HOW TO FEEL

Fighting Fit

Stories and advice to encourage and empower.

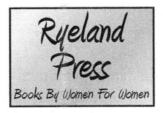

Ryeland
Press
Books By Women For Women

A RYELAND PRESS BOOK

By

JENNIE HOSKINS & SUSANNE GARNETT

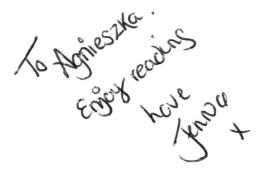

To Agnieszka.
Enjoy reading
love
Jenna x

HOW TO FEEL Fighting fit

Published by Ryeland Press.

Please note that this book is written using standard British English spelling and grammar.

Cataloging information:
ISBN 978-1-916927-03-2

Credits:
Cover Design: Chris Garnett. Canva
Illustrations: Susanne Garnett
Production Design: Karen D. Badger, Badger Bliss Books Manuscript Servicing

Acknowledgments

Many thanks to our book producer Karen Badger of Badger Bliss Books for turning this story into something publishable and working so fast and brilliantly to format and design the print and eBook.

Many thanks to our friends, beta readers, and reviewers who gave us great advice and kept us focused.

A special thanks must go to the women who have shared their personal stories in short testimonies which we have placed at the end of chapters.

Several of these stories talk of huge personal challenges and may be harrowing to read. We are so grateful for the candour and bravery you have shown in sharing your stories, which have inspired us, and which will inspire others who read the book.

Dedication

To women everywhere who live under despotic regimes and abusive regimes. Sisters, there are far too many of you. May our planet change for the better soon, so liberation comes to all.

Disclaimer

The authors are not medical professionals and do not claim to have specialist knowledge. None of the information or advice contained in this book is intended as a substitute for professional medical advice and should not be taken as prescriptive.

Readers should make their own decisions about how to use the book. As with any change of lifestyle, nutrition, or exercise regime, it is always advised to consult your doctor before beginning. By participating, you assume all risks and liabilities associated with the information or suggestions contained within the book.

Table of Contents:

Appendices:

Introduction

First of all, who are we?

We're two friends, twenty-five years apart in age, who met three years ago when Jennie met Susanne at our local fitness centre. Jennie was running a boxing and martial arts class, and Susanne, who had tried a whole range of sports and found she was hopeless at them all, decided to have a go at boxing. COVID-19 and other life events had kept her away from any real fitness program for the previous couple of years.

From then, it seemed a good idea to take some private sessions to catch up with the rest of the class, whose average age was about twenty-six, including several seriously fit guys and young women. We began to talk while Susanne stopped to catch her breath, and pointed out to Jennie the impossibility of doing star jumps when she hadn't taken both feet off the ground together for years, and so we made friends.

Susanne writes for a living, and Jennie trains people in fitness, so it's a partnership that seems right for this purpose, which is to encourage and support all women to lead fitter, happier, healthier lives. Of course, being fit doesn't guarantee happiness, but on the other hand, feeling unwell and unfit certainly can make you pretty darn miserable.

So, this is us:

Jennie Hoskins (2nd Dan Black Belt) is a professional fitness coach, specialising in Combat Sports, Krav Maga (Self Defence) Boxing, and kickboxing. Jennie writes more of her personal story at the end of Chapter 12.

Susanne Garnett is a writer, retired lecturer, charity director and grants assessor, with degrees in History, Theology, Social Psychology, and Adult Education. She has more than forty years of experience working with people all over the world to improve their lives by organising self-help groups in literacy, numeracy, and economic empowerment, life skills, and motivational training.

What's this book about?

Together we've decided to write a book of encouragement for every woman who would like to get fitter and feel better about herself and her health.

This book aims to support anyone who reads it, to not only understand their physical, mental, and emotional needs a little better, but also to find ways to enjoy life more, feel less pain, and less boredom, and even be released from addictive behaviors, whether they concern drink, drugs, food or negative relationships.

It's our blueprint for feeling, doing, and getting better, in body, mind, and spirit. The advice is our own, and it is important to say two things from the beginning.

Firstly, neither of us is medically qualified, nor we do claim to be health professionals. We would strongly advise anyone starting a course of exercise or making major lifestyle changes to consult a medical professional first, and to only work at a level that suits your age, weight, and level of fitness.

Secondly, how you use this book is entirely up to you. The ideas and suggestions in this book could be followed through a year or dipped into and used selectively.

Talking is all very well. This is an action-based manual though, and to get the most out of it, we invite you to do most of the 'work' yourself. Sorry about this, but you won't be alone. We'll be trying out all the suggestions ourselves, (especially Susanne, who needs to re-empower her life in many ways!)

This is a 'pump primer' book. More detailed exercise advice and workout suggestions will come in our next book, but this is designed to get readers feeling fighting fit. It aims to get the energy and happiness back into everyday activities, so that you can enjoy being alive.

The last few years have been hard for many people, and the future can look frightening, but we believe there is so much wonder and joy to be had, simply in being alive, so why not get ourselves fit enough to be able to enjoy it?

Here's to a great time together. Come and join the fun.

A question you might ask is 'Why is this book concentrating on *women*'s fitness only?'

There are two reasons. Firstly, there are many fitness manuals written by and aimed at men, and not all exercises or physical considerations apply to men and women in the same way.

Secondly, women's hormonal chemistry is very different from men's. The monthly cycle of menstruation and ovulation has a profound physical and mental effect on how we work as an organism, and the important change from childhood, through adult womanhood, to menopause, affects women in very specific ways.

Not every woman has the same life experience. We may have different sexual orientations. Many of us give birth, and many others do not, but our hormones and the effect they have on our body shape, chemistry, and aging process are the same. They are important and cannot be denied, and that is why we believe a book focusing on women's fitness is quite enough for now! We respect everyone's right to determine their gender, and to identify as they wish. We also respect women's right to privacy, and to feel safe. Bullying and violence against women should never be tolerated.

Sharing stories:

We want this book to be different in other ways from other fitness manuals. We knew it should be firmly based on the lives, knowledge, and wisdom of women, and before we even started planning and scoping the various sections in detail, we asked to hear from our potential readers.

We sent out questionnaires to more than a hundred women of our acquaintance, which mainly needed multiple choice answers or responses on a 1 to 10 basis of agreeing or not agreeing with a general statement. Those people we contacted were either clients of Jennie, friends of Susanne, and a range of contacts we had who were living mainly in the United Kingdom or the USA.

Our questionnaire wasn't very scientific, either in our choice of recipient, how we framed the questions, or how we analysed the answers! Nor did it set out to be a tightly controlled piece of research.

We wanted to get a feeling of what women's main concerns and attitudes were about their health and how they felt about fitness matters, especially after COVID-19 had run through both British and American societies with such devastation from 2020 to 2021.

More than sixty replies came back, for which we were grateful, and as we went through the answers to the survey, we were encouraged to see that the majority of respondents were trying their best to keep fit, but felt they should do more.

Some women who replied had been athletes in their youth, but had now completely given up team sports, and wanted to do some physical activity that would more easily fit in with busy lives.

About a quarter of our survey regularly used a gym or fitness center, and about a quarter never did.

Mental health concerns affected around half of the respondents, who said they worried about their health more since before COVID-19. Some expressed having increased anxiety since the pandemic, which had impacted their lives, and made them change how they lived, and how they viewed the future.

At the end of the questionnaire, we invited anybody who wished to do so, to write a little more on health matters, and we are pleased to include some of those very interesting and worthwhile testimonies at the end of our chapters here.

When we were choosing a title for the book, we played around with several phrases, e.g. *The Joy of Fitness, Keeping and Staying Fit, How to Get Fighting Fit,* but by the end, we hit on *How to Feel Fighting Fit.*

This was for a reason. In this book, we talk a lot about feelings, and also about the motivations needed to go into a gym or fitness environment.

This has come through talking to the women who answered the questionnaire, and who approached Jennie for fitness training.

Lots of women have multiple 'voices' in their heads that, whether intentionally or not, work to undermine their confidence. If this happens to you, this will de-motivate you, and make sure you don't reach your goals.

So even before we offer you menus, fitness plans, and a blueprint for exercise, we want to explore the feelings needed to embrace a healthy future.

Jennie is a specialist in combat arts training, and we met in one of her boxing classes, so the 'fighting' side of fitness training is one many women would enjoy and gain from. We hope you find this book an encouragement, and a starter to take you off the couch and maybe even through the doors of a gym. It is aimed at all ages.

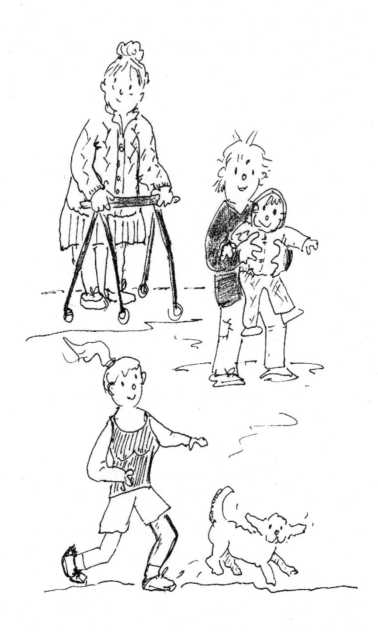

Chapter 1

Knowledge is Power

Susanne

Ever since early humans trekked north out of Africa to find a better life for themselves and their children, people have tried to understand the world and their place within it. We are still pondering on it, but who we are, and how we are meant to live is still a mystery to many of us.

Today, with all the advances in science and technology, and the fantastic skills and knowledge accumulated over the last million years, the world around us remains puzzling, as is the universe above our heads, and in so many cases, the workings of our minds and bodies! How can we care for something effectively if we don't know much about it, or how it works?

Just stop for a moment and visualise how your body would look on the inside if it was transparent.

Are you familiar with the *Bodytrax* analysis machines that can be found in many gyms these days? They are wonderful for giving you an instant reading about the density of your bones, the proportion of fat to muscle you have, where your fat is distributed, even how dehydrated you are, the amount of cholesterol furring up your arteries, and the measurement of your blood sugar.

It is often only when we hit middle age that these things interest us. It's then that internal twinges, aches, and pains remind us that our body might be telling us something. With the right kind of self-love, we can face the reality of our body as a functioning organism.

The harsh truth of what a body looks like inside, came home to me years ago, watching a televised autopsy of an obese woman who had died in her fifties and left her body for medical science. Every one of her organs was removed and its health or otherwise was explained in detail to the television audience.

It was a real-life version of *Silent Witness* and certainly was not easy to watch for everyone. But for me, it was an eye-opener. How we treat our bodies, for good or ill, has a direct visual result on our organs and this was made clear.

The woman's lungs were hardened and blackened by smoking, her liver had been nearly destroyed by cirrhosis, and layers of yellow fat enveloped all her internal organs. What was very touching was that she still had coloured nail polish on her fingertips, which only emphasised the poor soul's humanity.

In many cultures, including our own, there seems to be a traditional reluctance among ordinary people to understand how the human body works. Until recently even our means of reproduction was shrouded in mystery and lack of self-awareness.

This meant that in previous centuries 'well-brought-up' young women often went through their wedding ceremony without understanding how babies were made and what they should expect on their wedding night.

Those days are hopefully over, but cultural taboos run very deep. Only in 2023 did Wimbledon Tennis authorities relax the rule that women players must wear white shorts below, as well as white skirts or dresses above. Top female tennis players said how distracted they were on the court by having to worry about whether their menstrual bleeding would show through their clothes! This fundamental monthly reality facing half the world's population is still something ignored or found an embarrassing taboo by not only men but by far too many women as well.

Pain is also a great source of information about what has happened to us. It can carry the history of past injury throughout our lives. Broken ankles continue to twinge twenty years after the initial injury. Amputated limbs can still generate acute pain. One in four people will suffer some sort of chronic pain over the age of forty,

Senses such as hearing, eyesight, taste, and smell have their memory pathways. Covid has been proven often to have damaged the neuro pathways which give us our sense of taste and smell, as do other viruses, and some cancer therapies.

I grew sweet peas in 2021 and 2021 but couldn't smell the perfume of any of them! By the late summer of 2023, I could just about smell the strongest rose, but I still have a very poor sense of taste and smell. I have been told to keep smelling strong scents to re-educate my nose. Pineapple is said to be the most effective.

It is very important to learn as much as possible about your body. Do you even know your blood type? The aim is to understand and appreciate your body's strengths and weaknesses. In this way, you can be gentler on yourself or push yourself beyond what you normally try to do.

A few moments of meditation

Lie on the bed or a yoga mat in loose-fitting clothing and listen to what your body is saying to you. Tense and relax every part of it in turn. Take your time. Make the connection between your brain and your fingers, your toes, the small of your back, your hips. Say hello to each of them in turn, and then appreciate them for all they do for you. Fill them with positive love and understanding.

Feel the weight of your bones and of your breasts and belly. Accept them. They are you, just as much as your brain or heart is. Then think about each of your internal organs. If you're not quite sure where your liver or your kidneys are situated, look it up in a book.

This is the body you are going to nurture and nourish with good things from now on. This is your beloved physical self, who will carry your spirit forward into hopefully a long and fulfilling life.

You need to take care of it. You need to love it. You also need to guard it from harm and protect it from harmful addictions.

You may feel so relaxed by now that you nod off

> *to sleep for a few minutes. Your body isn't an automaton. It needs rest and replenishment. Above all, stop criticising it. There is something to love in everybody.*

When we're young we can get away with almost anything. Semi-starvation, junk food, weird diets, refusal to eat vegetables, drinking loads of high-sugar, high-caffeine energy drinks, abusing our liver with alcohol, and binge drinking, the list is endless. But somehow our body survives. We can bounce back and avoid killing ourselves. It may not be a pretty sight, throwing up at three a.m. after a night on the town, but at eighteen it probably won't kill us.

Many of us at some stage in our lives have treated our bodies like that. Youth makes you feel immortal, and usually at that age you don't have any real knowledge or understanding about the finer points of nutrition. Air-brushed fashion models are more likely to be a dominant influence on a young woman rather than a boring mother figure saying, "You should eat breakfast", or "Why don't you eat more vegetables?"

Part of the reason younger people can get away with being careless with their diets is that when we're young the rate of cellular breakdown and the body's power to regenerate is balanced. It is one of the wonders of human biology that we produce repair mechanisms that run along beside us and repair the damage we can do to our poor bodies by poor nutrition.

But at forty-eight, fifty-eight, or sixty-eight, eating poorly might very well be seriously life-threatening. As we mature, our bodies respond differently. They don't repair themselves so easily.

Our bodies tell us, *"Hey, not cool! I don't like what you're doing here. I need nourishment, not poison. I need food that will sustain me, build up my muscles and keep me in good shape, give me a happy stomach and a super-efficient digestion system.*

"What I don't want are hangovers, blinding headaches, nausea, pounding in my ears, insomnia, and mood swings. Please give me less fatty and sugar-heavy foods and salt, but instead, more water, not colas and high caffeine energy drinks!"

Fitness for a young person might be an option, but for anyone over thirty, it's essential. The good news of course is that it's never too late to turn things around. Good nutrition, coupled with muscle-strengthening exercises and flexibility training can reverse many painful conditions, notably Type2 Diabetes, and the stiffening and hardening of our organs and arteries.

As we age, the heart and the circulatory system

feel the strain more than the rest of our bodies. It's reckoned that we lose 1% of our aerobic flexibility and effectiveness every year.

Lungs can become less elastic if they are not exercised, and therefore less oxygen can get through to be transferred into the bloodstream. Blood vessels and the heart muscle can also harden and make it more difficult for the blood to circulate, hence the rise in blood pressure which is so much more common as one hits middle age.

This is a fact of life. It doesn't have to result in poor health, however, as long as we have a life plan to keep healthy. As we age the care and maintenance of these vital components, the unique configuration that makes us who we are becomes more of a consideration. Like it or not, the strength, flexibility, and speed given to us at the age of eighteen gradually need more and more help to stay in place.

Our minds, too, can grow stiff and set in a groove. Work, family responsibilities, and the normal wear and tear of an adult life can mean that by middle age, we can become negative and expect little joy in our lives.

Think of the bounding frolicking of young lambs compared to the solemn and slow walk of an adult sheep. Humans can be like that. We hear our grandchildren laughing and playing with their friends, rushing about simply for the fun of it, while we too often sit moaning about the world while we share a coffee or a tea with our equally sober friends.

When was the last time you laughed and laughed until your ribs hurt? Not recently? Probably not for quite a long time. Isn't that a shame?

So maybe now is the right time to be a grown-up and feed our bodies with what they need, to be a loving parent, as we would to any child in our care. No longer do we need to be reckless, taking unnecessary risks with our mortality.

It all comes down to loving ourselves and celebrating our bodies as wonderful creations and powerful machines. But to be a good parent means we need to exercise gentle discipline, not spoil ourselves, like a foolish caretaker rewarding a toddler with sweets all the time. Let's face it, one of the meanest things we can do to our bodies is make them carry a loaded rucksack full of potatoes around all the time.

But that's what we do if we are twenty pounds overweight. If you pick up a ten-kilo weight you might nearly buckle at the knees, yet you're asking your joints and bones to carry that constantly with you, all the time. If you do that, then you probably need to cultivate the muscles to cope with such an extra load, but maybe there is another way. Simply shift the weight and set down the rucksack!

Just think about it. Imagine our poor knees, hips, and ankles, the strain on our backs and hearts. We're not alone, either. This is the reality for over sixty percent of the adult population in the UK right now. Obesity, (what a fat-sounding word that is!) is the major health issue in the country, with twenty-nine percent of the population seriously overweight. Why have we ended up like this, and what can we do about it? Well, move more, obviously. The old mantra, "use it or lose it" kicks in here.

I know what you're probably thinking. *"Nag, nag, nag! Doesn't the woman know how hard I've tried to lose weight? Doesn't she understand how difficult it's been? Nothing works!"*

Of course, I understand. Now we know, let's look at ways in which we can improve our lives and feel fighting fit.

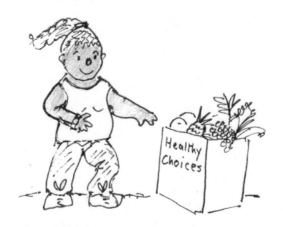

Chapter 2

Why bother to improve our fitness?

Jennie

We should all start to learn and educate ourselves about our well-being and fitness and learn to understand the difference between a marketing company that feeds our mind with false advertising and gimmick so-called diets, and real food, so we can start to shift our mindset to what and how we are looking to achieve.

Very often, our main aim or incentive to start a new habit, such as going to the gym, is weight loss. Losing weight to us in general is a euphemism for wanting to lose fat. Because fat makes us look and feel unhealthy and bigger than we wish to be.

But I think if we could change our mindset and split our goals into two different activities.

1) Losing Weight – Focus on Nutrition, and our meal choices.

2) Improving our fitness and wellbeing – Focus on being more active.

Why is it important to want to improve our fitness as well as focus on our nutrition?

Focusing on both our nutrition and physical activity is crucial for our overall health and well-being. The combination of a balanced diet and regular exercise provides numerous benefits that contribute to physical, mental, and emotional wellness.

As our bodies age and are part of our aging process, we need to focus even more on our well-being, and not take our health and mobility for granted. As we age, we will see a decline in our strength, flexibility, and overall vitality and this can be quite difficult to accept. This fitness decline can make even doing the simplest tasks quite challenging and can have a huge impact on own independence.

So, when people say to me "Oh, I am too old to start now" I tell them the older they are, the greater the need to improve fitness. I truly believe it's never too late to start something, and that if you feel inspired after reading our book you can achieve anything you truly put your mind to.

The NHS recommends we aim to achieve a minimum of 150 minutes of moderate-intensity exercise each week, or 75 minutes of vigorous-intensity activity each week. That's no more than twenty minutes a day, so should not be too difficult to start.

Aerobic Capacity

'Aerobic' means "with oxygen" and our ability to intake oxygen from the air around us. Our respiratory system extracts oxygen from the air and delivers it to our bloodstream, where it is used by our cells to produce energy.

As we age, our aerobic capacity generally tends to decline with age, due to various factors, including changes in muscle mass, heart function, and lung capacity and regular exercise can help mitigate some of this decline.

To help improve our aerobic capacity we need to train for at least twenty minutes at a pace that will raise our heart rate through activities such as power walking, jogging, dancing, rowing, cycling, boxing etc, etc.

Aerobic exercise also helps to train our hearts to pump blood around our body, so with each beat our heart pumps blood around, oxygen-rich blood. This process ensures that the body receives the oxygen and nutrients it needs and also removes waste products like carbon dioxide.

Our bodies are truly amazing, and we should learn to take responsibility for our own health. As we age it's so easy to sit down and to move less which our body loves. Yes, our bodies love doing nothing! We have to be strong-minded to get things done, just by reading the paragraph above you can see all the positive effects doing some daily exercise can have on your body.

To work out your Maximum Recommended Heart Rate

Subtract your age from 220 = your Max Heart Rate

We all have many ways to be able to measure personal data these days i.e. smart watches, heart rate monitors for training, etc. These devices help us monitor our movements by counting our steps, monitoring our sleep, etc.

Other problems affecting our ability to breathe properly include:

COPD – Chronic Obstruction Pulmonary Disease – the obstruction of our airflow, difficulty in breathing, and the ability to get oxygen into our lungs.

ASTHMA – This is a chronic condition causing inflammation and narrowing of our airways, which can lead to breathing conditioning.

PNEUMONIA – Inflammation of our lungs, caused by infection.

SLEEP APNEA – When your breathing stops and starts while you are sleeping. Sleep apnea is caused by your airways becoming relaxed and narrow whilst you sleep, and is linked to obesity and getting older. When we have disturbed sleep, this can then harm our daily lives.

Maintaining good respiratory health through regular exercise, avoiding smoking and vaping, and taking into consideration your environmental factors can help prevent some of the above conditions. If you have any medical conditions, you must check with your doctor before starting any exercise regime.

Not only does getting some regular exercise help your ability to breathe. which is a pretty important factor that we all need to live. but also participating in regular exercise can help to prevent other medical conditions such as **Diabetes Type 2**. This is a common condition that makes the level of sugar in the blood too high and is associated with various health complications, including heart disease, stroke, kidney disease, vision problems, and nerve damage.

It's one of the biggest health issues across the USA and Europe for people over forty and has to be taken very seriously. Managing blood sugar levels is essential to prevent these complications and maintain overall health. Physical well-being and efficiency help control your blood sugar levels and improve your

Insulin Sensitivity.

Why is Insulin Important?

Insulin is a hormone produced by the pancreas, and its primary function is to regulate blood sugar (glucose) levels in the body.

When we consume food, especially carbohydrates, our digestive system breaks down these carbohydrates into glucose. This glucose enters the bloodstream and causes a rise in blood sugar levels. In response, the pancreas releases insulin into the bloodstream. The food we eat has a significant impact on our blood sugar levels, as different types of foods are broken down into glucose at different rates. Glucose is a type of sugar that serves as the primary source of energy for our cells.

Carbohydrates have the most direct and immediate impact on our blood sugar levels. When you consume carbohydrates, whether from simple sugars or complex starches, they are broken down into glucose during digestion.

Complex carbohydrates found in whole grains, fruits, and vegetables are digested more slowly. Foods high in refined carbohydrates, such as white bread and sugary snacks, can cause a rapid increase in blood sugar levels.

What is Body Mass Index?

BMI = your weight in kilograms (pounds) divided by the square of your height. If your score is within the figures below, you can assess whether your weight is healthy or not.

Underweight = <18.5

Normal = 18.5 – 24.9

Overweight = 25 – 29.9

Obese = 30 – 34.9

Extremely Obese ≥ 35

But to be honest, I am not a fan of the BMI Index. It has also been criticised as being an inaccurate tool. This is because the BMI index only takes account of and measures your height and weight, so a person who has a high muscle mass and minimal body fat can have the same BMI as a person with obesity and a lot less muscle.

Osteoporosis

This is a condition that weakens our bones. A low calcium and vitamin D diet can increase your risk of Osteoporosis. This is more common in women than men and affects almost 20% (1 in 5) of women aged 50 and over at the time of menopause, as we experience a decrease in the hormone estrogen. We may not notice any symptoms until we break a bone.

Boxing and Kickboxing are proven to show these impact sports can help prevent bone loss' This is because whether you hit either pads or a heavy bag, the impact can create microfractures and result in your bones then growing stronger.

Depression and Anxiety

Depression is a common and serious mental health condition characterised by persistent feelings of sadness, hopelessness, and a lack of interest or pleasure in daily activities. It goes beyond normal fluctuations in mood and can significantly impact a person's ability to function in various aspects of life.

Anxiety is another common mental health disorder characterised by excessive worry, fear, and apprehension. While some level of anxiety is a normal stress response, anxiety disorders involve persistent and intense anxiety that interferes with daily functioning.

I would say as a coach, this is a huge factor in why you should start taking responsibility for your well-being, getting daily exercise / having a well-being program to follow.

Nearly everyone who trains with me says, "I exercise and turn up here basically because of the way I feel afterwards." This is especially true when those feel-good endorphins kick in, and they are feeling extremely proud of themselves.

Let's face it, not 100% of people look forward to stepping into the gym or a class. This in itself can be extremely daunting if you already are experiencing depression or anxiety.

Private training sessions are a great way to start,

with one-to-one coaching and a plan to work, to reach your personal goals. Find a trainer you like, someone who offers something you will enjoy doing, something you can set personal goals within, to improve every day, no matter how small or big the goals may be.

Chapter 3

Overfed but undernourished.

Susanne

Let's think about diet. In many ways our mouth is the riskiest area of the whole body when one considers what goes into it, and what comes out of it in terms of the things we say, and how we treat other people. Both are hugely important.

But let's consider:

What we eat

When we eat

How much we eat

How we eat.

All these aspects have changed quite dramatically in the last fifty years. If we analyse our eating habits and then put that knowledge, alongside all the fresh and useful knowledge available to us these days about the nutritional content of food, we might get somewhere to understand why so many people today are overweight.

Compare the diet of people in Great Britain in the

1950s with that of today.

Then, only a restricted range of food was available. In most families, they had a very simple range of foods. Spangles were about the only sweets on offer, and perhaps wine gums. The chocolate bars were very small, and a great occasional treat.

All meat was expensive, and a Sunday joint would be stretched through to the middle of the week. A free-range chicken would be a treat for Easter. Vegetables came straight from the garden or allotment, and the only salad dressing was the peppery salad cream squirted onto an otherwise undressed lettuce leaf.

Yes, it was rather boring, and not many of us would want to go back there. British food had a global reputation for being bad. But it kept people fit, and they were rarely overweight. There were few cafes and tea shops, and no such thing as ready meals.

I only remember having one very fat member of our extended family, Great Aunty Bessie, who weighed so much that she made my parents' Morris Minor car sink right down on one side if she sat down in it. (My mother would groan if she saw Bessie standing at the bus stop, and then felt obliged to offer her a lift.) Bessie told me she fell into fatness after she ate a whole Christmas pudding by herself, one she had made for the entire family of eight. But even she lived into her mid-seventies and was active to the end.

Most of the children I knew walked miles every day back and forth to school, up and down the steep hills of Gloucestershire, Yorkshire, or the Welsh valleys. We never had ice cream at home because most families didn't even have a fridge until the mid-nineteen sixties. If you had a dessert, like peaches and evaporated milk, you were told you had to have a slice of bread and butter with it. Cakes were always homemade, and therefore no more than a once-a-week treat.

There was no frozen food. Nearly every item eaten, milk, eggs, meat, and vegetables were fresh and consumed quickly. Potatoes were dug up just before they were cooked, and the main meal was usually lunch, a school dinner, with a light evening tea of a boiled egg, or bread and homemade jam. There was no such thing as margarine which tasted like butter. Margarine then, only came in a block that tasted like engine oil. Tinned goods had been invented a hundred years or more before of course, and lots of fruit and vegetables were bottled or canned at home as well, but we mainly ate fruit in season.

You may think this is a self-indulgent look back with rose-tinted glasses to an era when few people lived beyond the age of 70, so their time of retirement from an exhausting factory job might only be for five or six years. Life is generally so much better nowadays, in medical knowledge and practice, and in helpful medication and procedures, as well as supplements, we don't dispute that.

But the lessons that the war imposed on our parents and grandparents paid off in one important way. They proved that a frugal but nourishing diet, low in sugar and fat, and with limited amounts of natural unprocessed protein, unlimited vegetables and home-grown fruit, produced a healthy, slim population, capable of very active lives and sustained hard work, which was certainly needed to build up the country after the economic catastrophe of the second world war.

So, what should we eat to stay fit and improve our health?

"Five a day" is a mantra we hear regularly. Five portions of fruit and vegetables a day is considered the minimum needed for a healthy diet. It doesn't sound so much, not that difficult to achieve, surely? But sometimes, even if you have a large garden and bowls of fruit all around the kitchen, you may still get to the end of the day and know you haven't even consumed five portions of vegetables and fruit.

So, how about trying a new system? Eating by colours might be the answer. This is more fun, but you need to remember your rainbow for it to work.

Richard of York Gained Battles in Vain is the mnemonic many people learn to remember the order of rainbow colours, and that could help us *to* eat something Red, Orange, Yellow, Green, Blue, Indigo, and Purple, every day.

Here are some ideas to choose from:

Red: Tomatoes, radishes, raspberries, red peppers, red cabbage, strawberries, rhubarb, beetroot, cranberries, red apples, cherries, red onions, red grapefruit, canned kidney beans, plums.

Orange: Oranges, peaches, apricots, carrots, sweet potatoes, tangerines, butternut squash, pumpkin, baked beans, persimmons (Sharon fruit)

Yellow: Pineapple, grapefruits, yellow squash, swedes, yellow plums, Mirabelle plums, yellow peppers, bananas, sweet corn.

Green: Cabbages both green and savoy, kale, Cavolo Nero Italian kale, green grapes, broccoli, calabrese, lettuce, peas, runner beans, French beans, broad beans, watercress, Brussel sprouts, cucumbers, celery, endive, green peppers, sugar snap or mange-touts peas, courgettes, or zucchini marrows.

Blue: blueberries, blackcurrants.

Indigo/Purple: Purple sprouting broccoli, purple grapes, Victoria plums, damsons, aubergines, (egg-fruit), blackberries.

There's so much to choose from in these lists, and

they only contain produce commonly grown, not too expensive to buy, and easily available in the UK.

There are also all the lovely African and Asian vegetables to choose from, like papaya and mangos, which have some of the highest vitamin C content in the world.

Choosing brighter coloured fruit and vegetables and trying to get as wide a variety as possible isn't stupid, as the vitamin content is higher in many darker-coloured varieties.

We should have at least one serving of dark green leaves from the cabbage and broccoli family a day. Apart from the excellent roughage and vitamins they provide, they may also stave off the threat of dementia.

Fresh fruit is always preferable to dried, where the sugars are concentrated too much to be ideal. But frozen fruit is always available and much cheaper than the fresh alternative if the expense is a consideration.

A recent television programme about supermarket produce recently showed that it takes five fresh mangos to produce one small 200-gram packet of dried mangos. The mango farmer in Kenya who was interviewed for the show had never tasted the dried end-product, and luckily for him, he never needed to. He was surrounded by lovely fresh fruit growing on the trees on his farm.

It is good to eat greens, but unlike elephants and bulls, humans can't survive eating greenery alone. So, what else is essential to keep us fighting fit?

Protein:

This builds muscles and is vital for growing our bodies when they are young and repairing them as we grow older. About fifteen percent protein is the right proportion to be part of an adult diet, which will protect bones, muscle mass, and immunity.

There are nine amino acids that we need and are lucky because a wide choice of protein-rich foods provide them, both meat and vegetable-based.

Complete proteins, with all nine amino acids, can be found in fish, seafood, lean meat like chicken, and eggs. Egg-white is almost pure protein as it is designed to feed the growing chick as it develops out of the yolk. Luckily for us, all eggs, whether fertilised or not, provide the same nutritious little package.

A plant-based diet can also provide all the proteins needed by us, easily, if it includes soya and soya-based foods like tofu and tempeh. Millions of people across the world eat a plant-based diet, and by combining different protein-rich foods can enjoy a very tasty and varied menu without piling on calories or cholesterol. Legumes, like peas, beans of all sorts, lentils, and grains make excellent combinations.

We're now learning to love these meals. Before the introduction of the starchy potato into the British diet, (Thanks to Sir Walter Raleigh who brought some back they say from the new American colonies) pease porridge, made from dried peas, and bean stew with wheat or rye bread, made up the staple of most medieval people's winter food.

Today there is a huge range of cereals and legumes to choose from. We can produce meals based on rice, quinoa, buckwheat, barley, and freekeh, which is a fermented wheat much used in the Middle East.

On a choir trip to Italy a few years ago, treated to a supper of barley soup, which was simple but delicious. We were told it was a local specialty in the Perugia area of Umbria, where we were singing in some magnificent hill-top churches, and our whole choir had happy memories of the simple meal. Certainly, it must have helped the local people to run up and down those near vertical hills!

Carbohydrates:

A low-carb diet is popular among many people these days and can sometimes help reduce one's waistline in the short term, but it isn't carbs as such that are the problem. They are an essential part of our diet and provide sustained energy and support for the brain's function as well as keeping us alert and fulfilled without suffering low blood sugar.

No, the problem is **refined carbohydrates**, and let's face it, at the top of the list of villains are white sugar, corn syrup, and the other processed additives added to our diet. Sugar and its problems deserve a book all in themselves but the important point to remember is that **whole grains** of whatever sort, husk and all, are the answer when eating carbs.

A friend, trying to lose weight, was told "If it's white, don't take a bite" and that's not bad advice. We need the boring bits around the grain of rice, around the wheat, around the barley, and the bits that are hard to chew, like bran. When we add them, they add a crunch and a much deeper flavor to bread, pasta, rice, and other grains. They are essential to good digestion.

It's not only parrots and budgerigars who like millet if it's cooked properly. Eating seeds of all sorts can also add tremendously to our well-being. They are now sold in very useful packets of mixed seeds which can be sprinkled on nearly everything.

Why should we eat more whole grains? Because they contain the whole essence of the grain, including the fiber, and fiber is vital in maintaining a healthy gut. It prevents poisoning one's system with undigested and indigestible garbage. This is the one thing that the Western diet fails to achieve in a big way. We could all do with more fibre in our diet.

Mentioning the Unmentionable:

People in the West tend to think if they have a bowel movement, (or BM as nurses always call it) once a day, that is perfectly adequate, but other cultures regularly expect an easy BM after every meal and would regard anything less as constipation.

This makes sense. The digestive tract works best if it has a twice-daily rhythm. This means there is no strain involved, which can lead to very painful hemorrhoids and old detritus building up, increasing the risk of bowel cancer.

Constipation is a chronic complaint among many older people, and there is no need for it in most cases unless one is on strong painkillers and other medicines that slow down the evacuation.

It's usually down to the fact that we don't consume sufficient fruit and fiber, nor do we drink enough water. Dehydration is such an easy problem to fix.

Take a liter water bottle calibrated with a little section for every two hours through the day, to help drink regular small amounts of water with no fuss, and no bother. Often, we don't drink water because we simply forget to.

Lack of hydration can soon lead to brain fog, as well as the problems we've just been talking about, being chronically bunged up. As we age, common anti-inflammatories and painkillers are known for causing constipation but if we consciously increase our water intake every day the problem usually sorts itself out.

Both tea and coffee, while enjoyable, are diuretic and dehydrating, taking water out of the system and encouraging urination, so they don't act as a good alternative to water. Milk on the other hand is an effective rehydrator, and its calcium makes it a good drink, especially at bedtime.

When should we eat?

Intermittent fasting or limiting the hours in a day when we consume food is popular right now, made so by eminent writers and medical experts. Research has found that the risk of insulin resistance, leading to Type 2 Diabetes can be discouraged by not overloading our digestive system with too many meals.

A habit of eating early breakfasts, snacking throughout the day, and finally enjoying late suppers, does not give the digestive system enough time to recover. Instead, try limiting your food intake to eight or nine hours a day out of twenty-four. This may take some time to adjust to.

If you eat breakfast at eight a.m. and have an early dinner at five p.m., as many Americans do, this will achieve a better balance. But if you do not want to make such a radical move, then it is good advice always to stop eating after seven p.m. and certainly not to go to bed with a full stomach.

Many people enjoy two days a week of very light eating, with limited calories. Others eat fruit for all meals one day a week and eat 'normally' the rest of the time. There are many ways to fast, all of which result in a reduction in your weekly calorie intake. For most people that will be a good thing, and not cause any problems.

Fasting is natural and has been practised for health as well as religious reasons for thousands of years. It is not something to be scared about. The British prime minister, Rishi Sunak is said to always fast on a Monday. He stops eating on Sunday evening, resumes on Tuesday morning, and still maintains a focused and energetic working day throughout Monday!

How much we eat:

The average adult woman's stomach has the same capacity as a rounded cereal bowl, and our meals should come to about that size. The stomach can stretch, and in obese people, even after stomach stapling and other extreme solutions, it has been found that it can be distended again to an alarming size.

But our stomachs were designed to be the size they are for a reason. One bowlful size is enough to satisfy our appetites, but when eating gets out of control, the human brain seems to lose the ability to choose wisely and turn off the switch when nutrition is complete.

'Comfort eating' can play some nasty tricks on us. It starts as our friend but can end up as a tyrant, drawing us into an addiction that can seriously damage our health.

How we eat:

People eat differently in different parts of the world. Eating communally is the traditional way, sharing food from a common platter or bowl, sitting in a circle on the ground, sharing and talking. Some cultures invite one to eat in silence, meditative, but in the company of others.

The Western idea of a large family table with all generations gathered around it is still how we think of a traditional festive meal, but with smaller houses and isolated family units, this has become a rare treat.

Many of us these days treat our bodies as though they were cars needing to be refueled at a garage instead of civilised vessels to be treated graciously. Many families no longer sit at a table to eat, but snack on the sofa in front of a television or eat in front of a computer.

Not only is this bad for digestion, but it also encourages us to rush through a meal and eat without being mindful of every nourishing bite.

A well-decorated table, beautifully laid with clean cutlery, maybe a little bowl of flowers, and nice cloth or paper napkins can turn any meal into a special occasion. It also teaches children thoughtfulness and good manners.

***Sarah's story: Overcoming a huge challenge.**

My weight loss journey began in May 2018 when I visited the weight loss surgeon for the first time here in Finland. I had lost and gained so much prior but was scared of the gastric sleeve and bypass surgeries. However, I knew it was my best chance to shed the pounds. I weighed 416 pounds going in. I'm now at 286.

Before I could be approved for surgery I was told I had to lose about another 30 lbs. By surgery time I had lost about 37.

In March 2021 I had gastric sleeve surgery. After that I lost about 35lbs more. In March 2022 I had the revision to a bypass and have lost

---

another 25 since.

All told I've lost around 130 lbs. since my journey began. The process of low calorie and liquid diet wasn't easy prior to the surgeries, but I'm slowly still losing and I'm gaining muscle mass all the time. I feel like my body shape is changing and my desire to walk and move more has returned.

The difference is dramatic and often it feels like a dream that I actually did it. I was sad I couldn't do it on my own but so grateful for the tools I got from the surgeries.

I'm still a work in progress and learning but feeling better all the time. I'm only sorry I didn't start the journey sooner, but fear is a powerful thing and held me back from seeking surgery before.

Sarah

Chapter 4

Use it or Lose it. The Joy of Exercise

Susanne and Jennie

Good nutrition will help us stop getting fat. Regular, vigorous exercise will make us fit and definitely contribute towards reducing anxiety and sleeplessness.

We are, after all, still animals underneath all our fancy clothes and make-up, and as animals, we are designed to have good, strong skeletal muscles, a low regular heartbeat, a healthy gastro-abdominal system, and only carry as much weight as we need for the energy we expend, not to put too much pressure on our joints, or store fat as though we were going into hibernation.

Human beings are designed to move, not stick fast to a rock like a winkle. You only have to look at the thousands of people who regularly take part in full and half marathons around the world to see how our hundred centuries of evolution have not robbed us of this ability.

We may not need to chase an antelope across twenty miles of bush to get our dinner, but we still need to be able to push our supermarket trolleys around the aisles, pack and unpack forty pounds of groceries in and out of our cars, lift our children and help our elderly relatives in and out of the bath, and simply get out of bed every morning. We need to be able to move our bodies!

Aerobic Capacity

'Aerobic' means "with Oxygen" and our ability to intake Oxygen from the air around us. Our respiratory system extracts oxygen from the air and delivers it to our bloodstream, where it is used by our cells to produce energy. As we age, our aerobic capacity generally tends to decline with age, due to various factors, including changes in muscle mass, heart function, and lung capacity and regular exercise can help mitigate some of this decline.

To help improve our aerobic capacity we need to train for at least twenty minutes at a pace that will raise our heart rate through activities such as power walking, jogging, dancing, rowing, cycling, boxing etc, etc.

Aerobic exercise also helps to train our hearts to pump blood around our body, so with each beat our heart pumps blood around, oxygen-rich blood. This process ensures that the body receives the oxygen and nutrients it needs and also removes waste products like carbon dioxide.

Our bodies are truly amazing, and we should learn to take responsibility for our own health. As we age it's so easy to sit down and to move less which our body loves. Yes, our bodies love doing nothing! We have to be strong-minded to get things done, just by reading the paragraph above you can see all the positive effects doing some daily exercise can have on your body.

Some physical benefits of exercise - (If you still need convincing!)

- Enhanced flow of oxygen into the bloodstream and to the brain which helps us to concentrate and stay alert.
- Stimulated endorphin production. These are natural substances inside us which resemble morphine, and make us feel great.
- Improved circulation throughout the body which prevents blood clots, varicose veins, and piles.
- Improved digestion and easier absorption of food.
- Improved shedding of waste, through skin, lungs, bladder, and bowels.
- Lower cholesterol levels.
- Decreased blood pressure.

- Weight loss (when combined with healthy eating.)
- Improved blood sugar level.

Major mental health benefits can also be attributed to exercise. For example,

- Sleeping better.
- Feeling happier.
- Improved memory
- Reduced depression
- Greater control over anxiety
- Greater self-esteem.

So how out of shape are you? Here's a little checklist. Can you -

- Walk up a flight of stairs without feeling out of breath.
- Recover quickly from a climb of ten or more steep steps.
- Do short periods of exertion without exhausting yourself, like running for a bus.
- Lift and carry up to ten kilos of shopping easily from the car to the kitchen.
- Bend down and almost touch your toes.
- Undertake a team sport without feeling your muscles ache for days.

- Stand on one leg while you clean your teeth without falling over.
- Run at least a hundred meters without needing to stop.
- Sit on the ground and then get up under your own steam without having to ask someone else to help you.

If so, you have a reasonable foundation for undertaking an exercise programme, but always consult a health professional before embarking on new or more intense physical activity. If you cannot do these things, or find age has weakened your joints and muscles, then chair-based exercises are very good as well.

Now, you have to decide what exercise programme is right for you! There is no point in spending time and money on things that don't interest you. There are very many sorts of exercises to choose from, but they can be divided into some basic types.

Aerobic exercise is designed to reduce muscle tension and improve cardiovascular conditioning so that your circulatory system and delivers oxygen around your body more efficiently. It can also reduce stress and increase stamina.

Examples include brisk walking, running, cycling, (both outside, or on a stationary one), swimming, and dancing, e.g. guided routines like

Zumba dancing, or golf.

The idea behind aerobic exercise is to raise your heart rate to a level where it is a little stressed, make it work intensively at that level for a little while, and then let it relax.

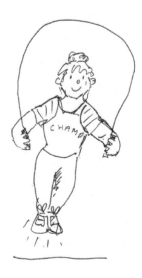

Here is a guidance table showing **maximum pulse rates** for various ages up to 70. Those over seventy should take professional advice.

Age	Pulse (heart) rate rise.
18-29	145-164
30-39	138 -156
40-49	130-148
50-59	122-140
60-69	127-132
70 plus.	Take medical advice.

Reflection by Judith: A Broken Hip

*In February 2003 it was my misfortune to fall &
break my left hip in a freak accident. Initially,
it was thought that I had badly damaged my left
knee because that was really painful, more than
my hip. However, after x-rays, it was
established that the fracture was in fact in my
left hip. I shall never know exactly what I did
except trip over on a pavement I had walked
along many times before & have since.*

*After the initial examination & x-rays at the
local hospital, I was transferred to a larger one
in our nearest city. There it was thought I
would have to have a partial hip replacement
but then for some reason, I was seen by a new
medical team & the Orthopaedic Consultant
said he would like to pin it.*

*This would mean a longer recovery period but
would work out for my good in the long run.
Eventually, if I needed a hip replacement, I
would be better off – or so I was told. To this
day, over 20 years later, I still have 3 pins in
my left hip & have not yet had to have a
replacement.*

*The recovery period was indeed quite lengthy: I
had ten days in hospital and was then sent
home with various aids including crutches, a
Zimmer frame & a wheelchair. I could not*

bend my left knee & was not allowed to weight bear for 6 weeks. However, I had to carry out specific exercises set by the physio three times a day and these proved crucial to my recovery.

After the initial 6 weeks, I could put my left foot to the ground & walk with crutches or sticks (usually the latter). Exercises continued. After some three & a half months I returned to work as a teacher and mainly walked around unaided. I didn't drive for three months.

There have been setbacks: I was prescribed a particular calcium tablet that caused stomach abscesses and I spent another period in hospital (the medication was stopped).

Too many steps/stairs on one holiday caused muscle damage and so for eighteen years I received treatment every 6 – 8 weeks from a chiropractor. I have had three of the latter, all excellent, and now only receive treatment infrequently. Walking & swimming are particularly beneficial; standing is not, nor yet sitting on a hard chair or pew for any length of time. I shouldn't kneel for long either.

I am now 70 years old & consider myself very fortunate to have received such good advice & treatment. I also feel blessed not to have had to have a hip replacement when several of my family & friends have had to do so. My right hip is good. I hope my story may encourage others.

Judith.

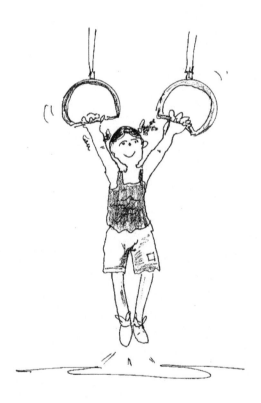

Chapter 5

The Great Outdoors

Susanne

If you can spend more time outdoors, breathing in fresh air, and experiencing the sensory joy of feeling a breeze, hearing birdsong, or the sound of wind whistling through the trees, you'll find it has a multitude of benefits for your health and well-being.

Here are just a few of the reasons to spend time outside.

1. You'll find it has a great impact on your energy levels. When you return to a task, you'll feel more energetic, more focused, and more clearheaded.

2. Taking a short stroll after a meal, rather than slumping down in front of the television will improve your digestion. If you decide to do this before eating dessert, it will be even better, because when you return, somehow the temptation of ending the meal with something calorie-dense and sweet will have disappeared.

For best digestion, it's good to be in a relaxed state, which walking achieves very easily.

3. It will increase your serotonin levels, and make you feel happier. Even a walk on a rainy day can do this, whether or not you choose to jump in muddy puddles!

Most of us have the basic equipment to start walking. After all, we started practising it from the age of one or two. It had many advantages over other activities. All you need are some decent walking shoes or trainers and there's no need to spend a fortune. You can walk in all weathers in the modern world, and Americans especially can be seen doing circuits around the shopping malls.

The arrival of exercise trackers and smart-watches a decade or so ago turned a simple movement into a measurable pace, and the 10,000 steps a day challenge became an obsessive compulsion with some people. That's the danger of any piece of kit or technology; it can turn something natural into an artificially strange activity.

Gyms all have treadmills, and step machines that mimic climbing up a steep hill add to the choice. You can quicken your pace from a gentle amble into a sprint at the press of a button, and again the desire to do better, run faster, and see your heartbeat rise, is good if done sensibly. But don't make it into a demanding compulsion.

If you can do more than walking, the "Couch Potato to Five K" program is a good one to join, it teaches you how to start slowly running for intervals in your walks and motivates you to continue. It may convince you that you won't die if you start a gentle jogging regime.

One positive phenomenon has been the development of weekly 5k park runs. These started as gatherings for serious runners but soon changed into a free-for-all with runners and walkers of all abilities joining in. There will be one near your home, so look it up and go along.

You need a brisk walk of about an hour covering three miles, to achieve aerobic conditioning, but even a twenty-minute walk with the dog twice a day is better than nothing. If your arms swing back and forth, it achieves something called "cross-lateral conditioning" which helps stimulate the right and left hemispheres of the brain. If it helps, invest in a set of Nordic walking poles to steady yourself as you walk.

Golf. This is gaining in popularity with women all the time, especially for those of us with the time and finances available to join a golf club. Some say it simply spoils a good walk, but the challenge of driving, pitching, chipping, and putting is irresistible to many, and even if you drive around the golf course in a motorised buggy, playing eighteen holes is bound to give you a good workout. Walking a course covers at least four miles, often far more.

I have tried to play golf, but my son says, "Mum, you move everything you should keep still, and keep still everything you should move." SG

Cycling. You never see a fat cyclist, do you? Cycling has many of the same benefits as jogging but puts less wear and tear on the joints. You need to cycle at more than fifteen miles an hour to achieve an aerobic effect though, and this takes time to achieve if you're a beginner, so take it steady at first and work up to that average speed. An hour's cycle ride three times a week, and you'll soon see results in your stamina and muscle strength.

If you want to cycle outdoors, there is the financial investment needed of a good bike, fitted to your height and build, a comfortable saddle, and a proper helmet. Avoid getting a racing bike, or a heavy-duty mountain bike, but look for a hybrid, general-purpose one. Bicycle engineering has improved dramatically over the last twenty years, and there is a perfect bike out there for everyone.

If you can meet up with a few friends on a Saturday or Sunday to take a gentle ride out for a couple of hours, you'll be surprised how much it can raise your spirits and reconnect you with the countryside.

Horse-riding (or if you're American, 'horseback riding') takes the joy of cycling to a higher plane still. In my life, some of my happiest moments have been while on the back of a horse, and if you can afford lessons, most reputable riding schools will take on beginners of every age. It is no coincidence why "Riding for the Disabled" groups have sprung up across the country, for the connection with a large animal, feeling higher than one would do normally, and sensing the constant gentle movement below one, all provide wonderful physical and mental therapy.

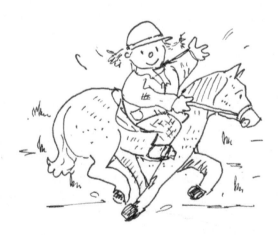

Riding a horse uses muscles no other sport seems to, and you'll be very stiff after your first lesson. But persevere, and you will soon experience the joy of going outside for a hack, or a trail ride in the States. Wild animals seem much less nervous of humans when they are on a horse, and the sounds, scents, and sights of the countryside seem more intense. It's an activity I would recommend to almost anyone.

Team sports, orienteering, ice skating. These are all fun and will get you fit as well. If you feel your exercise routine is in a rut, try something new. You may be surprised by how much you like a new sport, and how good you are at it.

Swimming. Some people enjoy a daily swim, even if they aren't very aquatic, and don't like putting their head underwater. A thirty-minute swim will improve flexibility and move every main muscle group. It is gentle exercise though, unless you are a champion swimmer, and by itself may not make you lose weight, but it will make you feel better and more relaxed.

The only downside to swimming in chilly climates is that it usually has to be done inside, in chlorinated swimming pools where the chemicals added to the water can irritate your skin and even your lungs. Always shower thoroughly after swimming in chlorinated water.

Swimming in the sea is wonderful (when the water is sewage-free!) and if you live somewhere warm enough to take a daily dip in the ocean, that can be one of the best activities in the world, for good physical and mental well-being. But again, shower afterwards in fresh water to remove the salt. Surfing or body boarding, for those skilled enough to enjoy it, takes ocean swimming to a new level.

Watch small children come out of school, and see how much and how joyfully they move. They will always skip instead of walk where they can. They'll jump up and run along walls, hop over the lines in the pavement, chase each other, and play tag. They are usually free and joyous. If we can maintain or regain that attitude that movement is natural, fun, and beneficial, we'll stay fighting fit for longer. So, let's go for it!

> ### *Reflection by Ellen*
>
> ### *The Benefits of a Brisk Walk:*
>
> *Along with other health and wellness activities, I discovered in recent years the physical and psychological benefits of engaging in a regular short walk of about 25-35 minutes at a moderate to brisk pace through a nearby residential neighborhood.*
>
> *I am fortunate to have this convenient natural resource available to me and have taken advantage of it (except when it's too rainy or cold!) since the early days of the COVID-19*

pandemic. Living in the U.S. Pacific Northwest city of Portland, Oregon, we are blessed with much natural greenery – including magnificent and majestic native Fir, Pine, Cedar, and Spruce trees. The homes in my walking path were clearly built in an area of old-growth forest, and many of those majestic tree resources were retained in the landscaping. Most trees are more than 250 feet tall, and many exceed 320 feet [note: include metric equivalents of height?].

In the ensuing weeks and months, my awe and appreciation of those specimens have grown. Stopping near the base of some of the gems, they genuinely appear to "soar to the heavens." It is truly an inspirational experience – a source of profound admiration, hope, and emotional renewal.

The ability to include this activity – or anything similar that increases one's "ancient bond with forests and nature" can indeed be a significant contribution to a woman's overall health and well-being. ,,, and (of course!) two of the physical health benefits of a regular brisk walk (which I do, on average, around 3-5 days per week) are cardiovascular -- and, importantly, strengthening of bone density (especially for older women -:)). My own most recent bone density scan (this past June) was normal and didn't detect any weaknesses!

And what do I substitute for outdoor walking when the weather is inclement' a frequent occurrence for eight or nine months of the year in our part of the country? My husband, who has mechanical and electrical engineering skills, has built a stationary exercise bicycle in his "man cave" room for us both to use! And while I pedal, he turns on his computer and acts as DJ as he plays our favourite popular music from the 1960's-80's! I rock out as I spin, and a great time is had by us both!"

Ellen Konrad, Portland, Oregon, USA
Resources:

Jensen, Edward C., Trees to Know in Oregon and Washington, Oregon State University Extension Service, December 2020, catalog.extension.oregonstate.edu.

Wohlleben, Peter, The Heartbeat of Trees: Embracing Our Ancient Bond with Forests and Nature, Greystone Books, 2021.

Chapter 6

Indoor Activities

Susanne and Jennie

It is said one expends 1500 calories a day simply by sleeping and eating. But who wants to do only that all day? Even if outdoor activities aren't for you there are plenty of indoor opportunities to get fighting fit.

Isometric exercises and weightlifting. These can rapidly build muscle mass and strength, but should always be undertaken with the supervision of a trainer or coach at the gym.

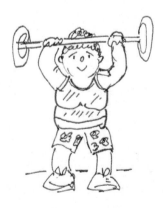

Be careful not to try to lift too much weight too soon. The variety of different machines within most gyms these days can provide a safe and monitored way to exercise every main muscle group.

As you progress you can add more resistance and gyms usually provide handy cards on which you can write down your circuit routine and record your progress. But the key is consistency. There's no point going once or even twice a month. Try to build in a routine of three to five times a week, for thirty to forty minutes at a time.

Body combat sports and oriental combat. These include Karate and Taekwondo, judo, boxing, and kickboxing, and have become much more popular in recent years. They provide a good combination of muscle development, flexibility, brain and body coordination, and a social element. They also provide a safe and effective way to get rid of pent-up frustration and aggression and diffuse excess adrenaline. There is also the important element of self-defence and self-protection.

Jennie writes:

From my experience as a coach, when anyone asks me what I teach, and I explain my main focus is to train for self-protection I will most of the time hear, "Oh I don't need that. I have never been attacked and don't want to learn how to become violent." Or "I'm too old to start that now. I have got to this age, and I'm fine."

But in my eye, my self-protection is not purely

about having the physical skills to be able to protect myself but the ability to protect my well-being, having the ability to feel good and function well. In addition, I want to be able to experience positive emotions such as happiness and contentment and to be able to develop my full potential in life and have a sense of purpose. Combat kickboxing offers you all that, and more.

How?

1. **It gives you confidence**. Not everyone is confident who walks through my door, and it can take some time even before they feel brave enough to attend their first session, I have done first sessions, as a consultation in a coffee shop, as nervous people can meet me in an environment, they feel happy in, and are not too overwhelmed with meeting me for the first time in a gym.

2. **Mental Health**. This is a massive aspect of training for me as a coach, as I see how it impacts on so many people's energy and sense of well-being. Many find it difficult even to get out of bed on a cold and wet winter's morning. (My alarm goes off at 5 a.m. six days a week, even if I do not need to go to work. I need this discipline to keep me on track, because I know if I roll over and snooze for another thirty minutes, I will wake

back up in a completely different mind frame.) Mental health is more affected by our physical state than we realise, which is why we focus on it in this book.

3. **Motor Skills**. These are the abilities that enable any individual to perform movements and tasks. We often take them for granted, but for people who have suffered traumatic injuries or who have been born with motor skill problems, simple tasks can become very complicated. These involve the coordination of one's brain, nerves, and muscles. They can be divided into two main categories:

   a. **Gross Motor Skills**. These are straightforward and give us the ability to run, jump, hop, clamber and climb, throw or kick a ball. They require our bodies to show physical strength, balance and co-ordination, and are dependent on the large muscle groups.

   b. **Fine Motor Skills**. Do you play the piano, sew on a button, write a letter, tie a bow? These all involve the use of fine motor skills which are the control and coordination of small muscles, particularly those in our hands and fingers. They can all be improved with practice.

Things we may take for granted, like using cutlery, cutting paper with scissors, and tying shoelaces, all have to be learned as young children. They can also be lost in later life through illness or injury. So, we need to keep every part of our bodies moving and strong to retain flexibility and strength. Combat sports are an excellent way to do this.

> ### *Reflection by Katie: Why I chose combat sports.*
>
> *I chose combat sports to help my physical and mental health.*
>
> *I also chose combat sports to learn valuable skills to help protect myself in situations where I could be at risk of harm.*
>
> *One of the reasons I wanted to learn combat sports is because when I was a young teenager I found myself in a situation where a man took me back to his home and sexually assaulted me at knifepoint.*
>
> *Back then the only thing I did to defend myself was scream and slap the man across the face.*
>
> *This did not help me get out of that situation, but the skills I have learned since then are more likely to help me protect myself if I ever find*

myself in a similar situation again.

Combat sports has also greatly improved my physical and mental health.

My personal trainer tailors my workouts to the areas I need to improve on, making my mobility much better.

This has improved my mental health as I can now do more and I have learnt how to eat and exercise   healthier.

Katie Bellamy.

Chapter 7

Mind over Matter

The Power of Our Minds in promoting good health and fitness.

Susanne

It's not only what we put into our mouths, or how often we get into our running shoes which determines how fit we are. The single most important dimension to achieving fitness goals is what is happening within our minds.

The connection between mind and body has long been established and known about for centuries, but even now, doctors and researchers are only just exploring the power of "Mind over matter" in affecting how our bodies respond. For example, a person under hypnosis, who is told a coin placed on their forearm is burning hot, will instantly develop blisters under it, even if the coin has just come out of a refrigerator!

On the other hand, a positive mental state full of

images of high-level fitness and achieving success and satisfaction, will not only promote healing, but it can also motivate you towards achieving energy like you've never known it, and keep you feeling and looking better.

Of course, by mind power alone, we can't add an inch to our height, or change the shape of our nose. But looked at holistically, how we THINK about ourselves, and our bodies, will have almost as important an effect on our well-being, as whether we have physically been exposed to disease, or caught a virus.

Many years ago, I read about a doctor in a prison camp who had nothing to give his patients except water. But every time he passed over a cup of water, he told them, "This is healing you. This will do you good." With only cold water, he was able to heal people from multiple serious conditions and restore them to health, keeping them alive until they were released from captivity.

This idea, that the mind can achieve anything it wants to, once considered the invention of what used to be called 'snake oil' salesmen, is today a respectable part of accepted medical opinion. There have been too many scientific studies to think otherwise.

Large-scale research projects held over many

years have demonstrated how negative emotions can exacerbate illness, and how having a positive attitude can help restore health much faster and more effectively than physical therapy and medication alone.

It's not a new idea that negative states of mind like anxiety or depression are important factors in the genesis of illnesses as widely different as diabetes, asthma, colitis, and disorders of the heart, but until recently the medical establishment paid little attention to the psychological components of those diseases. Now the relationship between the state of our mind and the ability of our body to protect us against illness is accepted everywhere.

One study in the USA of 900 graduates over 16 years, demonstrated that people who suffered feelings of isolation and had little sense of closeness to their parents as children had a significantly higher incidence of cancer than others.

Even more, sadly, it's been proven that those babies whose mothers suffer stress before they are even born have less ability to empathise with others and may even become sociopathic due to the excess of cortisol flooding into the placenta while they are in the womb. People who tend to experience anxiety, nervous tension, and anger under stress also have a higher incidence of coronary heart disease.

So, we must accept that our mind, the way we think about ourselves, and how we view our future, will strongly influence our fitness level and our recovery from illness. Blind tests with the use of placebos, whether fake drugs or even mock operations which have no power in themselves to heal, have shown that if a patient believes the intervention will do him or her good, then this can have a potent effect in healing.

Scientists are only beginning to penetrate the mystery of how placebos work, but they are beginning to discover specific ways in which thoughts and emotions influence the biochemistry of how we age and our health. This is exciting stuff indeed.

Endorphins and enkephalins

It hasn't been so many decades since biochemists first uncovered the existence of potent pituitary proteins and peptides such as endorphins and enkephalins, which can induce a state of pleasure in a body. They are produced as a result of experiencing positive emotions, and a direct link has been established between a person's expectation of health from a placebo and the biochemical changes that will bring it about.

Not only do these neurotransmitters serve as channels of communication within the brain and central nervous system, but they also link states of human consciousness to biochemical processes. Some activate immune responses and help protect us from illness, but they can also do other marvelous things, like improving our ability to learn, absorb and retain information.

Neurotransmitters have been shown to have remarkable antidepressant abilities or will intervene in some of our functions such as sleep, oxygen intake, and heart rate. The link between mind and body has never been more clearly understood, but there is still so much to learn.

The human mind is like a wonderful continent we are only just beginning to explore, and we are learning all the time.

So how do we achieve a 'super health' attitude in our minds? Is it that easy? Most of us, perhaps especially those who suffer from chronic conditions like arthritis, or Coeliac disease might understandably be very sceptical about the ability of the mind to cure physical conditions. However, let's think about it for a bit.

Our imagination is one of the most powerful tools for change we can find anywhere. We may not realise, but we use it all the time. We can imagine the best, or dwell on the worst scenarios. Our imagination operates for better or worse on our health, relationships and work, most of the time, unconsciously influencing how we view ourselves and our place in the world.

We continually tell ourselves things, but are they negative or positive? "Oh, I do feel tired. I look old. I'm frightened of getting cancer. I could never do that."

Block out the Negative Voices.

It's like we shut ourselves up in a castle of limitations. I was in my early twenties when I finished my first full-length novel, in response to a competition put out on the radio programme "Woman's Hour." There was a deadline of three months ahead, and the first prize would be serialisation of one's work as the book of the month on the programme.

I was a full-time mother of small children, so I had little time, but the idea inspired me to try, and I started to write a story, on a very small portable typewriter, mainly in the early mornings after my baby's first feed of the day, and before I had to prepare breakfast for the rest of the family.

I had a vision of a finished novel in my head, and that idea kept me plodding along until I had finished a respectable 50,000 words and had a manuscript I could send off to the BBC. I didn't win the first prize as the judges said my story wasn't quite exciting enough to make it to the top spot. But I was in the final shortlist, and they advised me to seek publication. This I did, and the first publishers to whom I sent it accepted it and offered me a three-book contract.

Since then, I have written twenty novels within different genres, but my goals were nearly scuppered for almost forty years by a casual comment from my mother, who merely said, "Oh, I hoped you'd write a proper, serious novel, not just a romance story." I let myself listen to her negative feedback and stupidly avoided any more fiction writing for three decades!

I only tell this story to show how the things that feed our imagination, for good or ill, can alter the whole course of our lives.

When you write you are at the mercy of reviewers and if you let it, one negative one-star review can undo all the good that ten five-star reviews can give. That's why some of my fellow writers never read their reviews at all. It's easier though to ignore the 'trolls' on the internet, who tell us we're rubbish, than do the same with the criticisms from inside our heads, with which we punish ourselves unnecessarily.

There is an old story of two wolves living inside us. One is kind, positive, brave, happy, and successful. The other is mean, unkind, pessimistic, bitter, and cowardly. The wolf who will triumph to run our life is the one we feed and pay attention to.

Using the imagery of the wolves, most of us tend to live on at least two levels. We have positive images of ourselves, bouncing with energy, young-looking, and successful which we can allow to play through our mind. This is the image we try to display to the world.

Underneath though it's a different state of affairs. If we're honest with ourselves we are also plagued by doubts and inadequacies more often than not. We may fear failure and we perhaps have a sense of personal hopelessness or powerlessness.

The latter comes from thinking or assuming that the human being is basically powerless to change anything and we're really only pawns in the game of life.

Making effective use of your mind power is to bring these two levels together to soften all those nagging self-doubts and strengthen your ability to make use of the imagination.

Think of what positive changes you want to achieve, and this will put you far ahead in the journey to great health. The way to do this is quite simple and doesn't involve weird psychic powers or airy-fairy practices.

Visualisation – A most powerful tool.

It is based on creating a strong image in your mind of what being fighting fit is going to look like for you. But it needs constant reinforcing, so let your mind play on these images, when you're stuck in traffic or waiting for a bus, relaxing, exercising or doing the ironing.

Keep at it, and you will find you'll change your mind set on what you can achieve, and how great the future looks. The stronger and clearer your positive image is, the more detailed and personalised you can make your fantasies about your future success, the more likely are they to stop being fantasy and become part of your everyday reality.

There are lots of books and expensive courses offered to teach you how to do this, but it doesn't need the brains of a rocket scientist, or spending £1000, to change your mindset and outlook.

Okay, by looking up at the moon, you may not instantly become a rocket scientist, but you might decide it worthwhile to sharpen up your maths skills, and also look up at the moon, the stars, and the whole universe more often than staring down into the gutter in despair.

Here are some suggestions for strengthening your positive mindset.

- Following on from the "Love yourself" meditation in Chapter 1, imagine how things would look if you were to reach your full physical and mental potential. Harness your inner goddess.

- Learn not to be phased by changes all around you, steering a steady course forward. In life, change is inevitable, so why not concentrate on the task at hand and don't fret too much about the future?

- Aim high. You can be top of whatever class you want to join. No horse ever won a race by lolloping along in the middle of the pack. Try to be the best you can be.

- On the other hand, stop being paralysed by perfectionism. Think of the Islamic teaching that only the Divine is perfect. Humans do and should make the odd mistake.

- Look outwards, not inwards. Be a good friend and expect people to be friendly and supportive in return.

- Don't fret about the small stuff, like trivial physical problems.

- Laugh when you can, as often as you can, especially at yourself. Have a sense of humour about your foibles and follies. Don't take yourself too seriously.

- When you wake every morning, assume it will be a good day when you will feel great, and everything will go well.
- Before you go to sleep at night, count the good things that have happened that day. Take them with you into your dreams.
- Never "let the sun go down on your wrath."

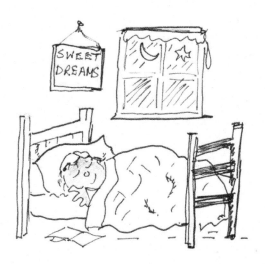

Chapter 8

The Benefits of having a Personal Trainer/Coach

Jennie

When you are looking for a Personal Trainer, remember you are going to be willing to Invest your time and money in it, so it is key to find one you know will be able to coach you for your personal development, not only for weight loss, which is the number one reason why the majority of people start their search for a Personal Trainer. If you find the correct personal trainer, they will be able to offer you so much more than this.

Personal trainers are certified professionals with a deep understanding of exercise science, nutrition, and fitness principles. They can design a customised workout and nutrition plan tailored to your specific goals, body type, and fitness level, ensuring maximum effectiveness and safety.

Having a customised workout devised to your own personal goals is key, or you can attend as many gym sessions or attend as many classes as you desire but you wouldn't see a progression towards your goal. Don't get me wrong, any kind of exercise and social interaction is a step in the right direction. But if you have a specific goal, that's when I would advise researching Personal Trainers whether in person or online.

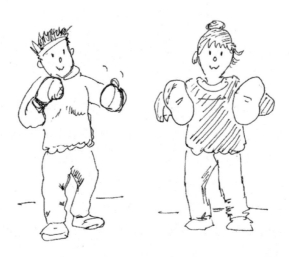

Whether you're aiming to lose weight, build muscle, improve cardiovascular fitness, or achieve any other fitness goal, a personal trainer can create a structured plan to help you reach your objectives faster and more efficiently.

Personal trainers consider your individual needs, preferences, and limitations. They can adapt exercises and routines to suit your unique circumstances, making the journey more enjoyable and sustainable.

Having a scheduled appointment with a personal

trainer can help you stay committed to your fitness routine. The encouragement, guidance, and support they provide can be crucial for staying on track, especially during moments of low motivation.

Performing exercises with correct form is essential to prevent injuries and ensure that you're targeting the right muscles. A personal trainer can teach you proper technique, monitor your form, and make necessary adjustments to prevent potential problems.

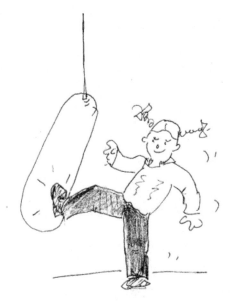

Personal trainers can introduce a variety of exercises and training methods to keep your workouts interesting and challenging. They can also adjust the intensity and complexity of your workouts as you progress, preventing plateaus and ensuring continuous improvement.

A personal trainer can design efficient workouts that maximise results within a shorter time frame. This can be particularly beneficial for individuals with busy schedules.

Working with a personal trainer can help you learn about exercise, nutrition, and healthy habits. This knowledge empowers you to make informed choices even when you're not training with them.

Reflection by A.B.

My name is AB. My childhood wasn't the greatest. I lost my father when I was six years old. This marked me and I didn't realise how much it affected me until my twenties. My grandad became the father figure in my life but unfortunately, I lost him in 2004.

When I was around twelve years old, I was abused and beaten by my mum's boyfriend on a daily basis. At the beginning, I was locking myself in the bathroom when I could hear my mum being beaten. I was so scared but I wanted to help her so I decided to stand up for us but I was too weak, so I sometimes took the beatings instead of her. This abusive period lasted around

---

four years.

I needed a lot of therapy to get through the trauma from my earlier life but after a period of intense therapy, I was able to learn more about myself and I was ready to learn something new. I chose to learn about self-defense.

It took me a while to find someone with whom I clicked until I found Jennie. She gave me so much strength and I'm so grateful for it. With all the techniques she teaches she makes me feel so strong and unstoppable. I will never be that scared little girl ever again locked in the bathroom. I'm capable of standing up for myself.

I think every woman needs to feel safe and strong. I found that self-defense training helped me to feel so much more confident and able to defend myself. I believe that every woman should consider learning some kind of self-defense.

Chapter 9

A Good Night's Sleep

Susanne

There is no doubt about it; the modern world isn't good at sleeping. Look at the TV weather map of Europe - the lights sparkle out into the universe across the whole continent, and in North America, urban parts of Asia, and around the rim of Australia even, it's the same.

When did we all decide to leave the lights on all night? It never used to be like that. It's as though we are all trying to defy the laws of nature and stay awake twenty-four-seven. Only in a few isolated places in the UK, in the Highlands or north Northumbria, central Wales, is it possible to see the stars. My friend has built his own observatory high in the hills north of Machynlleth. I was in Gambia in 2004, far from any town before I saw the full glory of the heavens. We deprive ourselves of so much.

On the corner of the road by my house, the streetlights shine all night, and it's a very quiet country lane with minimal late-night traffic. Animals and birds must be suffering as well. Even the trees and flowers are having a hard time dropping off. It seems crazy madness to me, to waste so much power, and I commend campaigners who are arguing against such massive waste of electricity.

According to US medical experts, adults need at least seven hours of uninterrupted sleep for our brains and bodies to function at optimum levels. Anything less than that can result in the neural connectors, vital to sustain our ability to memorise and to learn, failing to do their jobs.

Children of course need much more peaceful sleep. A baby should sleep between twelve and sixteen hours a day. Primary school children need at least nine hours. The earliest, most ancient children's songs were lullabies for a reason.

But how many children get a good night's sleep? I'm amazed at the number of parents who keep their children up all the time, and fill the house with television programs, games, and music until midnight. No wonder they fall asleep at school and can't concentrate.

A recent USA survey found that 40% of American adults survive on less than six hours of sleep a night. And this can result in coronary heart disease, obesity, high blood pressure, and quite a few more of the ten most serious human diseases. Sleep deprivation also results in cell inflammation and a compromised immune system.

So how do we get a good night's sleep? Well, the NHS website has plenty of good straightforward advice. We'd do worse than start there. But I have twelve golden rules for perfect sleep, based partly on the teaching of Doctor Hansaji Yogendra, the sagacious head of the Yoga Institute in India.

On her YouTube channel, she stresses that sleep disorders disrupt the parasympathetic nervous system, resulting in a circle of stress, which in itself causes insomnia. Check her out!

My version of how to achieve restful sleep which means you wake up energetic and joyful is to take a holistic view.

So maybe we need to look at:

Where we sleep

How we prepare for Sleep

How we lie down to sleep

How we eat and drink before sleep

How we control our anxieties and worries, to ease our mind into sleep

How we stay asleep.

So, let's think about all these things, and then see

if our own night-time routine and environment correspond to the best practice.

Where we sleep:

Sleep experts who run labs so have to get their volunteers off to sleep, say that the ideal temperature of a bedroom should be between 65 degrees to 72 degrees. It's better to sleep in a cool room with a warm cover on the bed, than in a hot bedroom under a thin sheet.

The room also needs to be dark, which is why one should either turn off all electrical appliances, chargers, computers, etc., or leave them outside the bedroom altogether. I used to have an alarm clock which shot a bright blue light with the time onto the ceiling. That had to go! If your room is too bright, invest in blackout blinds, or even cheaper, buy an eye mask.

Many of us sleep with our phones beside our beds. Another bad idea. Try to be daring and **leave your phone in another room** on charge. Leave it unanswered between 10 pm and 7 am. The world will not cease to turn if you switch it off.

Pets can also be big sleep disruptors. At the risk of upsetting lots of people, I would advise against having your dog or cat sleep in the same room, let alone on the bed. But anyone who has been woken up by a cat pawing their face at 5 am knows what it means.

How We Prepare For Sleep:

Begin to calm things down an hour before your normal bedtime. If you have trouble sleeping, don't turn on an action film on TV after 9 pm. It will overstimulate you, and probably keep you up too late.

Falling asleep in the chair in front of the telly, and then lying awake half the night later is a common problem for the over fifties. So, try to stay alert in the evening, and save your rest for later.

A late-night short walk around the garden, or down to the end of the block and back, possibly with your dog, for twenty minutes or so, is a good practice, and helps you take in some oxygen before you sleep.

Establishing a little routine, like putting out the milk bottles, locking up, cleaning your teeth, and hanging up your clothes, all helps prepare the unconscious mind for sleep. Many people like to read in bed, but others find this too stimulating. Some prefer to play one Sudoku puzzle, which is nonverbal and clears the brain of verbal clutter.

It is said a drop in body temperature is good for sleep, and one way to achieve that is to take a hot shower. In the West, we like to shower in the morning.

In Asia, in Korea, for example, it is far more common to shower the last thing before bed and to lie down clean and relaxed. A shower or a bath can also help our muscles relax into a very peaceful pre-sleep state.

How We Eat Before Sleep:

Don't eat a heavy meal any later than three to four hours before sleeping. A little drink of hot milk however, perhaps with a teaspoon of turmeric in it, and another small spoonful of honey, however, is a good nightcap.

Chocolate or cocoa can be very stimulating, as both the sugar and the caffeine can agitate the nervous system.

Don't take caffeine later than lunchtime unless you want to be up at 3 a.m. It is better to stick to de-caff coffee or herb tea like mint or liquorice.

Delving into the freezer for a midnight snack of ice cream probably means that your nutrition has been seriously compromised during the day. Expecting to enjoy a peaceful night's sleep on a full stomach full of alcohol or sugar is a pipe dream.

How do we control our anxieties and worries, to ease our minds into sleep?

Some people find a short time of prayer,

reflection, or meditation before sleep, dwelling on the events of the day and laying them to rest, is one good way to stop the brain racing about like a hamster in a cage.

An old tradition was to kneel by the bed and say some formulaic prayers. You might want to start a journal. At night write down three or four things you are grateful for that happened during the day, things that went better than expected, unexpected little triumphs or joys, for example.

Early the following morning, maybe over an early drink, you might look at the list again, and then write down three different things you'd like to achieve that day, and visualise them happening. Managing your thoughts can channel them in the right direction, and help prevent nightmares ruining your sleep. Your brain is a very cooperative partner and will often do what you tell it, once you've trained it.

(I kept a record for a long time in my journal about how much sunshine there had been in the day. Even in rainy old Britain, I was astonished to see just how many days in the year did contain at least an hour of blue sky and sunshine. The weather was brighter than I had remembered!)

How We Can Stay Asleep.

If you find yourself waking up at a ridiculously

early hour, or even sometimes only minutes after falling asleep, then running through a little relaxation meditation can help. Start with your toes, and flex and tighten each muscle group in turn, then let your body fall into a relaxed state again.

Do it slowly, breathing in on a slow count of four and out on a slow count of eight, and you will probably find you are asleep before your stretching and relaxing reach your shoulders.

I also find a little 'sounds' app, which plays the sound of rain falling, or ocean waves lapping against a shore, nearly always sends me to sleep within the ten minutes I set it to last for.

One reason of course for waking in the night is the need to wee. This also gets annoying more frequently as we age, for both men and women. An obvious solution you might think would be to avoid drinking too much in the evening, but an oversensitive bladder and poor pelvic floor muscles can cause a night-timed need to urinate regardless of when you last took a long drink.

A good workout should include dynamic pelvic floor exercises, including strengthening the inner thighs. We tend to leak as we age, especially if we cough or laugh, run or jump. So, strengthening the lower abdominal muscles and the inner vaginal tissues can help prevent this happening. Being overweight will put more pressure on the bladder of course, as will constipation, which is another reason to drink plenty of water.

Thoroughly hydrate yourself during the day and you'll be fine. It is very important to keep hydrated, and many women are more dehydrated than they imagine.

Many mothers find it especially hard to sleep like a log once they have had children. A small part of the brain remains alert for a child's cry or distress for the rest of one's life. But we don't need to stay awake like a night-shift worker. Gracefully retire and allow yourself the luxury of a good night's sleep. You deserve it, and your body will soon tell you if it isn't getting enough rest.

If you have a chronic problem with sleep, of course, consult your doctor, or ask at the pharmacy for a gentle herbal sleep aid, which might tide you over a difficult patch. Times of insomnia through personal trauma, bereavement or physical illness may of course need to be treated with some medical assistance so don't be ashamed to ask for help.

We spend a third of our lives asleep, and good sleep solves big problems. Some physical conditions do cause sufferers to feel chronic exhaustion, and they never wake refreshed and full of energy. But if this isn't you, then give thanks, and help your body achieve what it needs to stay fit and well.

Chapter 10

Happiness

Susanne

Introduction:

Taking the ideas about mind over matter from the last chapter, ask yourself, "If we're concentrating on getting fighting fit, does it matter if we're feeling happy or not?"

Well, yes, it does. How we feel affects our entire well-being.

What is happiness?

A more scientific word for happiness, used these days by psychologists is 'subjective well-being'. This is a fancy term, but it does pinpoint the two main ideas behind what we know as happiness. Firstly, it's not a 'one-size fits all' idea, and secondly, along with great happiness, we will probably go through great sadness. It's called being alive.

Just as we all might have different tastes in food or favourite colours from other people, we also each experience happiness very differently. It's subjective.

But on the other hand, there are some common reasons for happiness, which go right across all societies, and even some we share with animals. Think of a dog or cat gently snoozing on a hearthrug, with its paws running along in a dream, as though they are chasing a mouse or a rabbit. Don't say they're not having a happy dream! Or on waking, see how a dog will madly jump up and down and wag its tail immediately it sees its owner coming home.

Our body's strength, our energy, the way we deal with stress or difficult times like bereavement, and the health of our internal organs and nervous system are all deeply improved if we have a fundamental sense of well-being and happiness.

I also believe that there is such a thing as a broken heart when all happiness and hope of future happiness is taken from us. People do die from it.

So, while many of the topics mentioned below in this chapter are dealt with in more detail elsewhere in the book, we think a discussion of happiness, and the various ways to promote within ourselves is well worth including.

The History of Happiness:

Trying to achieve happiness is not a new idea. The Greek philosopher, Aristotle, (born 384 B.C.E.) discussed it at length in his written works, and because he was always keen on categorisation, taught that it could be divided into four distinct levels, or types, as follows. Here they are:

1. Achieving immediate gratification. - e.g. Grabbing the last slice of chocolate cake on the plate and consuming it.
2. Comparing present achievement with previous lack of success. – e.g. Passing an exam well, or learning to swim.
3. Making a positive contribution to the well-being of others - e.g. Volunteering at an animal shelter or fostering children, or something much more minor, like opening the door for someone, or giving up one's seat for an older person or someone who has difficulty standing.
4. Achieving fulfilment in life. e.g. having a long and happy emotional partnership or seeing one's children grow up to be well and happy.
5. Of course, one might add romantic or ardent love for another human being as a fifth source of happiness, even though it may soon lead to tears!

The world's religions have spent a great deal of time discussing happiness in one form or another. Essentially a widely held view among all religions is that anything one might strive for on earth will not make one truly happy forever.

In the Judeo-Christian tradition, earthly ambition, or even anxiety about where the next meal was coming from would not lead to happiness. *"Consider the lilies of the field; they toil not neither do they spin, yet Solomon in all his glory was not arrayed as one of those."* This is very similar to Buddhist teaching, which advises us to rise above all earthly ambition or attachment.

Aristotle taught his pupils something similar, that achieving wisdom and understanding and living according to one's values, was the only true road to happiness.

Current research:

There have been many recent research projects into happiness, including those by major universities, like Harvard, and the University of British Columbia, but these projects have failed to pin down any exact formula to achieve it. As we said before, one key finding is that each person's happiness is unique to them.

But there are some interesting overall findings one might use.

Having Hope:

This is a core feeling shared by happy people. They are optimistic. Even if things are bad now, they will get better.

Have you heard the little story about a boy who was always happy, to the great annoyance of his employers? They did all they could to make him depressed, including telling him to clear out an enormous stable full of animal dung. But he set about the task with gusto and whistled as he worked. "Why are you so cheerful?" demanded his boss. "Well," said the boy, "With all this manure about, there must be a pony nearby!"

So, the anticipation of new things, getting a new job, or a new house, and seeing a positive dynamic in your life does provide happiness. But discovering you are expecting a longed-for baby, the research found, gives a greater sense of joy, than the ongoing pregnancy.

Looking forward, with positive plans, and taking action to achieve them is one way to happiness. Abraham Lincoln is quoted as saying "The best way to predict your future is to create it."

The key seems to be in **self-empowerment, and having a positive self-image,** which gives you the necessary energy to create more happiness for yourself and those around you.

In South Korea, a study found that **possessing spirituality** came top of people's list of what made them happy, followed by good, strong social relationships.

In Australia, another study found that bringing up positive memories and dwelling on them rather than always recalling past resentments and perceived slights increased people's sense of joy and contentment, and made them happy.

Not always the richest or most successful.

I have found, during my work across the world in very poor communities, that it is never the richest who are the happiest. Indeed, it's been proved over and over again that it isn't the case.

Being granted a £5 loan to buy one sack of maize made one woman I met in Kenya incredibly happy. With it, she started a market stall, pulled her family out of dire poverty, supported her injured husband and his second, previously hidden family, and survived life in one of the worst slums in Africa.

I know of someone else, on the other hand, who rose almost to the top of his profession, to fame, and status, even appointed to a seat in the House of Lords, and who had control over many hundreds of people. But because he wasn't promoted even further, to the very top job in the country, he sank into great bitterness, fuelled by alcohol and fury at being passed over.

This has been documented and is called "Arrival Fallacy". It highlights what the great philosophers

Jennie Hoskins-Susanne Garnett

and religious teachers say, that personal ambition and a wish to succeed, while they can be positive drivers in your life, do not lead to lasting happiness or lasting contentment, with what you have.

It is often seen in celebrities and high achievers. When they sometimes reach the top of their profession, instead of joy, they are often surprised to be filled with a sense of anticlimax and even despair.

"Is this all there is?" is a common question they ask. And then, if they aren't helped to deal with it, highly successful people can end up with dependency on drugs or alcohol to mask real depression.

On a much smaller scale novelists say that when they finish writing a book, there's a sense of anti-climax and the adrenalin seems to drain away once they've written "The End". They can feel really low, even depressed for a few days.

If you recognise this in yourself, if you achieve something great, or finish a big work project, you can anticipate this happening and know how to deal with it. Switch off the computer, get out into the sunshine, phone a friend, and make a date to meet and catch up. Clean the house!

Aristotle said much the same thing. He said we should always look for the "Golden Mean", the balancing line between deficiency and excess. Not too little or too much, but just enough.

That is perhaps why our world seems so stressed and globally anxious right now, as most people in the world try to manage on far too little, while the gap between rich and poor has stretched out more than at any time in human history. One man can have more money and resources than whole countries today.

Habits of Happiness.

So, what can we do to find and capture the elusive butterfly of happiness? The NHS and other public information websites have lots of good advice, which I have whittled down to some simple ideas.

The acronym MAJOR provides a peg on which to hang these suggestions.

M - Meaning in Life. This seems to be a global foundation for happiness. Long-lived and productive communities all across the world have been proven to have a spirituality that gives meaning to their lives. This doesn't have to be through one religion or another or the same spirituality. But, if one has a sense of being alive for a reason, with a strong set of values that one follows through by living in accordance to them, it promotes happiness.

Living with a sense of gratitude for life itself follows this, and on a daily basis, if one can rise with a sense of gratitude and at night lie down with a list of all the things one is grateful for, then it's a good and positive way to frame the day.

A - Accomplishment. Unhappy people often have poor self-esteem, believing they aren't any good at anything, that they're not good-looking, that no one will want to spend time with them, and that they will never amount to anything. Sometimes these negative thoughts are pushed into them by bad parents, abusive spouses, or bullying bosses, but they can really drag people down, and make them very unhappy.

Classic coping strategies if you feel like this might mean you hide away, avoid social situations, and try to avoid challenges at which you might fail. The avoidance tactic can help in the short term, but it often backfires, especially if one seeks comfort by over-eating, drinking alcohol, or using drugs.

The answer lies in pushing back on those beliefs you have developed about yourself. Write down at least six good things you know about yourself and keep repeating them. Write them on paper and stick them on the fridge or where you clean your teeth. Ask those who live with or near you to tell you positive things about yourself, and you'll be surprised by how many things they come up with.

We all need affirmation and a sense of accomplishment. The next thing to do is to write down every day a list of things you've achieved that day. They can be small, simple things, like cleaning the kitchen, walking the dog a few hundred yards further than normal, or picking and arranging a small bunch of flowers.

If you need bucking up, join a local class to learn a new skill. You'll make friends that way. I know someone who completely lacked confidence with computers, so she signed up for classes at her local library. They were free, and the atmosphere was very gentle and non-threatening. She did so well that the librarians asked if she would volunteer once a week to act as a champion of the training program to help those who were less confident to make similar progress! Now she does this every Wednesday and it's become a highlight of her week.

J – Joy. What a lovely word that is! And how rarely do we experience it as sober side adults? When was the last time you laughed yourself silly? Do you remember a time when you were in your teens when everything seemed funny, and you had a fit of the giggles at the slightest thing? It's almost as though when we're young we can gamble and laugh and chase about like lambs in a field, just for the joy of it, but as we get old, we turn into grumpy old sheep with our heads down and only concentrate on munching through the field of grass.

Joy can be life-giving. It can be deep and restorative, and they've proved laughter is good for the whole body, producing those endorphins we all need. This is why people turn to alcohol I suppose, because there is nothing more boring than being the only sober person at a party, when everyone else seems a bit tiddly.

I get my joy in different ways. Being out in nature invariably gives me joy, and the beauty of the English countryside always profoundly reaches me. I once lived by the sea at Filey in North Yorkshire, so every night I fell asleep with the sound of the sea through my windows, and that gave me a sense of great joy and connection with the wider mysteries of nature and our natural world.

Walking dogs down the six miles of golden sands and seeing the gannets diving into the water for fish wasn't so bad either.

I also find gardening very relaxing, and now often ease myself into the day by walking through the garden at dawn, listening to the hens and cockerels chuntering and chirruping to each other, and also catching the birdsong concert from the surrounding trees.

In September long skeins of pink-footed geese begin to arrive from the Arctic Circle to congregate in the skies above us. Watching them fly in formation and listening to them call to each other is profoundly joyful.

I am very lucky to live in the countryside and to have a garden where I can grow a range of vegetables.

But when I worked in an office, I grew cherry tomatoes along my windowsill and used to go outside during the lunch break to sit by the river and watch the dippers and kingfishers. Little capsules of happiness like that, provide happy memories that are life-sustaining.

Classical music is another source of joy for many, both listening and singing and even playing instruments can be profoundly joyful. I was especially inspired by the young soloist French horn player in the BBC Proms concerts in 2023 who had no arms, so he played the Mozart horn concertos with his left foot.

O – Others. So often our happiness depends on others. But we can take more control of how we interact with them and be proactive in making our relationships positive and joyful.

Back in the 1930s, Dale Carnegie wrote a book called, *"How to make friends and influence people."* It became an international best-seller and was often seen as the bible for salesmen and people who needed to make a good impression. It was easy to poke fun at it. But within it, there is much good sense.

Dale Carnegie grasped the truth that if you want people to like you, then you have to like them. You can find something good to say about anyone, and few people do not respond positively to a small, genuine compliment, not just blather, but a sign that you have acknowledged them, and seen something good about them.

He tells the story of meeting a Catholic nun, and wondering how he could compliment her without giving offense. Then he hit on the right note. "Sister," he said, "What a beautiful speaking voice you have!" How she beamed!

Speaking of nuns, this is a little story about how we often find it much harder to receive positive affirmations than give them.

I used to have a faded, blue sweatshirt with writing across its front which read "Two hugs for survival, six hugs for maintenance, and twelve hugs for growth". Once, when I was leading an assertiveness workshop for women in a convent, an elderly nun passed me in the corridor, read my sweatshirt, and almost cried, "No, no that's impossible! I can't give out anymore. I can't hug anyone else. It's too much to ask!"

I said as gently as I could, "Sister, but it's not about you needing to hug other people, it's the number of hugs you deserve to receive in a day."

She looked at me in astonishment. She'd been taught that her needs were quite unimportant and that she didn't deserve and shouldn't seek to be loved and cherished. Of course, I had to. I gave her a warm hug, and she gradually relaxed in my arms and squeezed me back in return. "Where did you buy that?" she asked. "Can anyone order one?"

Being kind to others is a way of being kind to yourself. The Dalai Llama says that all true religion should come down to these two words, "Be Kind." And he should know.

But you don't always have to rely on others. You can also be kind to yourself, and self-care can be an important part of every week's routine. We all take showers these days, but to sink into a long hot bath with scented bubbles and maybe a candle or two lit on the edge can be a wonderful treat. You might even paint your toenails while you're at it!

This leads us to the final letter in the acronym.

R – Relaxation. If you are stressed, anxious, miserable, or angry, it's very hard to relax. But learning to relax completely can restore happiness better than almost anything else.

We mentioned animals sleeping earlier. Well, there is nothing more relaxed than a sleeping cat, draped along a window seat or over the back of a sofa. Or think of dozing seals on a rocky outcrop next to the pounding waves of the Pacific Ocean. (Okay, so the mother seals relax, while the males fight, yes, we know.)

We humans are mammals, not so unlike cats, dogs, or seals, but in today's hectic world, we seem to have lost the ability to relax. Many people find it very difficult to sleep at night, let alone take forty winks during the day.

But you don't need to completely fall asleep to be relaxed. Even in the busiest of households, it should be possible for you to sometimes take a warm, leisurely bath, maybe with the door locked against inquisitive and demanding children. You could also sit down with friends to watch a football match on the TV or meet for coffee. Taking ten minutes outside in the fresh air can also help us relax.

At our local gym, most mornings, after an early swim, a group of friends tends to gather for coffee in the lounge, to exchange news and have a chat over the newspapers, and just relax for twenty minutes or so before we go off to work or do other duties. Friendship between women is one of the greatest gifts in the world.

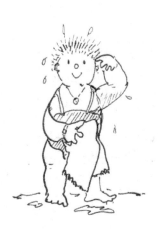

Breathing techniques, simply inhaling and exhaling to the count of five can relax one instantly, and reduce one's blood pressure. It's not hard, but so often we almost forget how to do it!

One sensible suggestion to help one's brain relax is to turn off anything electronic for as long as you can cope without them. This may only be for 30 minutes, (in which case you really might have a problem!) But try not to take your phone to bed with you. Switch off your computer for at least one day a week. Read a 'proper' book instead of an electronic reader now and then.

A routine of taking a 'Sabbath' from the electronic demands of the world can be very relaxing. This is a good theory and practice (though one I find hard to do!.SG)

So **MAJOR** might be a word to give basic help in seeking that balance that leads to lasting happiness. If it doesn't help you, then invent your own.

The important thing is to know we all deserve to be happy. It should be a natural part of our life, just as sometimes it is right to be sad, or angry, or regretful.

Happy people attract others. So does a smiling person. The physical act of smiling has been proven to make you feel better, just a little, but enough. How bad is that? Why not smile at yourself today?

Reflection by Heather: Living with Addison's Disease

After two years of sickness, two weeks being bedridden & serious weight loss, Addison's Disease was finally diagnosed late in 1979. I was thirty-one years of age. My adrenal glands were not working – not producing the hormones that are essential for everyday life. Daily drugs were now required for life, and with the consultant hammering on the hospital bed - 'You must never be without these tablets'.

Other questions came to mind: my mother asked – 'Can she have children?' I asked - 'Can I drink alcohol?' The responses came quickly. 'One with medical attention & one in moderation'.

I learned I was a 'listed disease' – i.e. I was entitled to free prescriptions & was advised to wear a medical bracelet.

I decided that this condition would not define me, so I attended all medical appointments alone, and within one year of diagnosis, I flew a long haul to Canada, obtained a higher-level teaching post in another Local Authority, completed a degree course at the local university and bought my own house. Addison's Disease did not prevent me from obtaining a mortgage, all necessary insurance, or being able to purchase or drive a car.

I had a busy career teaching Geography – organising field trips to the East Yorkshire coast, climbing hills in the Lake District, and camping with teenagers in Norfolk. I worked in educational administration, became a school Inspector & a Diocesan Director of Education. These full-time jobs were always stressful and without adrenalin, apart from in tablet form, I was often extra tired and questioned whether I could fulfill my roles to the highest standards I expected of myself. I had been told that I should contact a doctor if I needed to take additional drugs to manage a particularly stressful situation, but this proved to be totally impractical, & I learned to break tablets in half and take them as I felt necessary. I didn't appear to come to any harm.

Other medical conditions needed substantial attention to the amount of medication one was taking – the common cold; dental work; COVID-19; non-Hodgkins Lymphoma; two hip replacements; polyps in the bowel and pneumonia. Medical professionals had input into the administration of medication whenever I was hospitalised, Student doctors regularly came to talk to me about the condition as it was something they had read about but had never met anyone who had Addison's Disease and led a full life.

My religious faith was something I had grown up with, questioned when I was diagnosed with Addison's Disease, and stood back from for about ten years. Yes, I did ask the question 'Why Me?' However, another house move, a return to live closer to family & friends, and a re-engagement with a local church brought me back to belief in God and this is part of my everyday life.

Leisure time included membership of a local choir for over 40 years, with weekly rehearsals, and concerts locally and further afield in the UK and at Cathedrals in Europe. I studied as an undergraduate and then undertook a master's degree alongside working full time and eventually retiring early to care for elderly and vulnerable parents who reached their nineties. Their support over the years was crucial in ensuring I survived this far.

The theatre, cinema, meals out with friends, visits to London particularly, holidays in the UK and in Canada & the USA have been important activities throughout all these years.

Addison's Disease - an unusual medical condition to live with and one does not come across others in the same situation very often. Fortunately, medical professionals have been very understanding of the condition and in some cases, we have learned together as years have gone by.

It has not defined me but has been the backcloth of life against which every other decision has been taken. Time for medication!

Heather Morris September 2023

Chapter 11

Dealing with Anxiety

Susanne

Firstly, it is important to stress that we are not qualified or trained psychologists, and cannot provide the level of information you might need if your anxiety problems are serious. All we can give here is a summary of the main symptoms, and make some tried and tested suggestions for coping.

I used to have a Snoopy calendar with a January cartoon where Charlie Brown looked at the days ahead and said, *"Just checking what I have to dread this week."* I'm sure you've known that feeling, at some time in your life, for at least some of the time, if not constantly.

It's thought that more than fifteen percent of the population in the UK suffer from anxiety to the level at which it impacts our everyday routine and makes us less able to enjoy life. So, if you are part of the 15% or one in every six or seven people, then know you are not alone.

People have always been anxious. Life for human beings has always involved avoiding or fleeing danger and coping with profound grief and fear as part of life, as well as the normal everyday ups and downs and mood swings.

However, several things have made the problem of anxiety worse in the twenty-first century. We have built an extremely sophisticated globalised news media, so the tragedy of a bus crash in Italy comes straight through our living room, as does an earthquake in Morocco, a flood in Bangladesh, or a drought in East Africa. We are bombarded with negative news, about which we feel powerless to alter or react against in any meaningful or positive way.

We're also faced with a plethora of choices everywhere we turn, what to eat, what to wear, which car to choose, what lipstick to wear, and this demanding focus on diversity of choices is pumped into our eyes and ears, by a relentless advertising industry.

The creators of the adverts don't know us or what we like or don't like, but now they are using artificial intelligence to stalk us across the internet and push advertising designed just for us. Social media is funded by it.

This is so commonplace we've become used to it. But it can still sting. A friend did some online research into nursing homes in her area which might eventually suit her aged mother, only to be bombarded by advertisements from funeral directors and bereavement services. All too much!

A lack of time and space to digest all the external stimuli thrown in our direction makes this worse. The pace of life is forever getting more frenetic and impossible to slow down.

Even pedestrians who could once stroll through a city between shopping or appointments are now encouraged to jump on electric scooters, whizzing through the streets and narrowly avoiding disaster at every corner.

Other factors in the rise of anxiety might include, the falling away of adherence to the traditional religions which provided a bedrock of faith and confidence in the teachings of religion, eating too much processed food with a high reliance on sugar and stimulants, universal access to very cheap alcohol, caffeine and narcotics, and working practices which mean that one's home can no longer represent a safe sanctuary away from professional stress and a boss's demands.

Then of course we have the ubiquitous smart phone, which monitors our every move, and buzzes in our ears constantly, asking us to respond to every idea, every inane request, every picture of someone else's sandwich. No wonder we risk being in a permanent state of nervous over-stimulation and anxiety.

But to our generation, especially affecting young people and children, the new and frightening idea that we might all be wiped out by a pandemic has been added as another worry. The dread of another disease similar to the plagues of the past has joined our list of things to make us anxious. Our world is getting smaller, and viruses travel everywhere.

Finally, and most universal of all, we have the most global of all threats, rising temperatures, and unpredictably violent weather which are already proving the climate-change scientists right. Our grandchildren will face challenges we have yet to understand, or even know enough about to prevent.

***

Anxiety can show itself in a range of ways, including insomnia, obsessive-compulsive behaviour, panic attacks, avoidance techniques, bursts of anger and fury, and torpor, and can lead to serious mental health problems, and most serious of all, the development of long-term degenerative diseases.

Bad news, eh?

So, what can we do about it, if any of these symptoms impact our own lives? We can do much to help ourselves. But above all, we need to improve our ability to withstand all this cumulative stress and strengthen our immune system.

There are some basic points I would make.

Firstly, nothing can be improved unless we take a holistic approach, as we've stressed throughout this book. Physical, mental, spiritual, creative, - all aspects of our minds and bodies have to work together for wellness and happiness.

Secondly, we cannot work in the present without understanding how much the past has impacted on us. It has created our reactions to events, our mindset, whether we are optimistic or pessimistic for example, whether we dwell on sad memories, or have suffered trauma which means our bodies go into flight or fight mode too quickly and inappropriately.

The past is like an ocean on which we all swim. Those who have been taught to swim well keep afloat and reach their destination, but some are in danger of letting the past drown them. Mindfulness and living in the moment is a good thing, but you ignore your past at your peril. We are the sum total of all our previous minutes, for good or bad.

Thirdly, women, because of our hormonal makeup, are often deeply affected by our menstrual cycles and the life changes that affect us. We talk about this in more detail later in the book, but our internal nervous system can be affected and make us much more tense and anxious at some stages in our lives than at others. The old jokes about "time of the month" do no justice to the challenges many women face, but mood swings are a physical reality and can lead to intense anxiety over small things that later present no obstacles.

Anxiety can appear in many different ways and at different levels. One might feel it as a child starting at a new school, where you tremble with fear, your stomach seems to be tied up in knots, and you have an urgent need to dash to the toilet. An actor suffering from stage fright might feel his heart beginning to thump, or her palms grow clammy with sweat before walking out in front of the audience.

I suffer from fear of heights and know I might feel faint when facing an exposed precipice. This happened to me once when walking on Striding Edge in the Lake District, and I had to retreat in ignominy. Standing on the top of the Liver Building in Liverpool recently had a similar result. It seemed irrational, but I could not look straight down without feeling I would faint or fall over.

Other fears and phobias are easier to cure. As a child, I was taught to imitate my mother who always screamed if a moth came into a room to flutter around the lampshades, and screamed harder still if a mouse ran across the kitchen. Now I would be delighted to see more moths flutter around the outside lamps at night. There are far too few of them!

We also cured my mother's phobia about mice when my ten-year-old son had a pet mouse, and she watched with fascination how it ate seeds and nuts with its little hands and tried to reach out through the bars of its cage.

These are what one might call situational fears or anxiety, like fear of flying for example, and can be helped by gentle exposure to the situation in a supportive way. But what happens when our fear of flying prevents us from ever going on a plane, and we suffer anticipatory panic at the very thought of it? Then we might need professional help because there are lots of ways out there to find support and therapy.

One acute symptom of anxiety is a spontaneous panic attack, defined when you show four or more of the following symptoms:

- Shortness of breath, and/or difficulty breathing
- Heart palpations – rapid or irregular heartbeat
- Sweating
- Nausea or the urgent need to open one's bowels
- Trembling, shaking or dizziness
- Acute sense of dislocation from reality, of being outside one's body.
- Choking
- Fear of death
- The sense of something crawling up one's spine.

These symptoms may all be frightening at the time, but the important thing to remember is that they are *symptoms* of the panic attack, and they will subside quite soon after the panic attack peaks and then calms. Many people suffer from them and eventually learn to distinguish between a panic attack and other purely physical causes of the symptoms. They can be a one-off occurrence, come in a cluster and then subside, or be a regular unwelcome intrusion into one's life.

If you experience panic attacks, seek medical advice. But there are other, less impactful ways of dealing with milder anxiety or general lowness of spirits. The following strategies have been proven to help in many cases. The key is to take positive action, to do something, rather than let anxiety overwhelm you.

1. **Breathe!** So simple an idea, but when we are scared, we tend to hold our breath, rather than use it to settle our feelings of panic. Deep, abdominal breathing, slowing down one's breathing, and taking long, slow breaths to the count of four, do two important things. It blocks the main symptoms of the fight or flight response, increased heart rate, and tightness in the chest. If you can simply breathe slowly in and out for three to four minutes, it will calm you down and clear your mind. Practising this type of breathing

exercise several times a day will teach you how it feels, and help you build it into your routine. Stand by an open window and get that oxygen into your bloodstream. Breathing is good for you, and all animals!

2. **Speak health to yourself**. Say affirming truths, rather than negative lies to yourself. Words have great power, and the way our inner voice talks to us can make a huge difference. But we can control that voice, and make it more optimistic, sweeter, and kinder to ourselves. Imagine you have to give a presentation. From "I won't be able to cope. I'll make a fool of myself, and everyone will laugh at me" to "I have prepared well. I know this material and I have nothing to fear," isn't so hard a progression. Simply taking a deep breath and saying, "And relax!" to ourselves when we feel tension rising, is often enough to transform the situation.

3. **Move around** or engage in some physical activity. If you are feeling anxious, achieving some small task like washing up the dishes, or straightening a few cushions might be enough to 'take your mind off' what's worrying you.

4. **Talk to a friend** on the phone, someone who knows you well and won't either fuss or offer unhelpful advice. We all have someone in our life who knows and loves us well enough to understand. If you don't though, be brave enough

to ask the universe to send you someone. They will arrive before very long.

5. **Stay in the moment**. This is what mindfulness means, not imagining future catastrophes, or dwelling on past disasters. Feel the moment, think how good it is to be alive, to hear the birds, or the traffic, to smell a sweet cologne or your favourite furniture polish! We are all given multiple senses and they can support us by helping us focus on the now, rather than the then. We can change neither the past nor the future, but we can control this moment and our reaction to it.

6. **Experience something pleasurable**. No, don't rush for the cookie jar, but why not ask your partner to give you a little loving, even some sex, which is the best relaxant in the world if you are in the mood? Live alone? Take a warm shower or a bath and treat yourself to a favourite body wash or shower gel. Pick up the phone and order a healthy, special takeaway. Re-read a favourite book, or watch something funny on the television.

7. **Get mad, not miserable. It's an** interesting truth that anger and anxiety can't live together in one's mind or body. If you are angry, then anxiety can't get through. So, if something has upset you, then get that anger out! Sit in the parked car with the windows shut, and have a good scream, or if you're home, feel free to rage and swear as well. Tell it as it is. If screaming isn't enough, then

don't be ashamed to punch that pillow, or whack the bed or the couch with a cricket or baseball bat.

Think of how small children can throw terrific tantrums at the drop of a hat, and hit out at anything within reach. Then they calm down and feel better. You can do the same. Anger is natural, and like a kettle whistling when it comes up to the boil, we all need to let it out somehow.

Just don't take it out on your family or loved ones. Deal with it yourself. Kick a ball against a wall. If you have a garden, go and pull out some weeds. Chop wood even.

Abraham Lincoln said he spent the whole of his youth with an axe in his hands, living out in the backwoods, and all that hard work probably helped him stay calm and courageous in his troubled years as President.

People who were brought up in violent households are often too frightened ever to show anger themselves as adults, burying it. But left unresolved, rightful anger can turn into anxiety and self-hatred. What happened to you as a child won't happen again. You were right to feel anger. Let it out. You can even enjoy whacking those memories away.

Anxiety is an unwelcome presence in many of our lives. Some people do seem to have been born with anxiety hotwired into their DNA, but it doesn't have to be like that for most of us. Physical activity, calming foods, good friends, and a calendar on the wall with some pleasurable things to look forward to, can all help us cope. There is no shame at all in seeking a trained counsellor or therapist, either.

Life is for living, for loving, and for having some fun. So, let's go and do that.

Reflections by Linda

As a survivor of sexual abuse since the age of 7 years I have had negative thoughts and complex issues regarding my body image for most of my life.

I have struggled with eating disorders throughout most of my young adult life and well into middle age.

Sixteen years ago, I experienced systematic bullying by a senior female manager which led to over-eating/comfort eating.

As the weight piled on, the smart, close-fitting suits became looser, floaty dresses to disguise the weight gain. From my normal weight of 8 stone 7 lbs, I gradually reached 13 stone 2 lbs which left me feeling constantly exhausted, sluggish, and increasingly miserable with my

---

body image.

One day, when I realised that I was avoiding looking at myself in the mirror because of how disgusted I was with how overweight I had become, I decided that I needed to take up some form of regular exercise. I joined a local Leisure Club where I was advised to lose weight using a combination of exercise and healthy eating, rather than by drastic dieting, to keep the weight off more easily and effectively, long term.

Over two years, I lost just over 4.5 stone and have managed to keep the weight off by daily exercise and healthy eating six days each week over the last fourteen years.

For me, regular exercise is now a complete mind set and, whilst I enjoy my one day "off" each week, my body always feels ready to get back into the routine after it.

Last year, my beloved husband of nearly forty years, died after a long illness, knocking my self-confidence and exercise/healthy eating regime out of the ballpark. With the support and encouragement of good friends, however, I managed to return to the Leisure Club three weeks after his death where the re-established routine of exercise, peer support, and camaraderie gradually began to restore some sense of "normality" and purpose to my world.

Throughout my life, I have been aware that I have numerous obsessive-compulsive personality traits – not least of which in relation to my rigorously controlled eating habits and strict exercise discipline.

During the last few months of my husband's life, it felt as though exercise was the only area of my life over which I still had some control. This resulted in me pushing myself far harder than I really felt capable of / wanted to simply because I feared that, if I didn't do my full routine, I would lose the last element of control that I still had in my life and that was a terrifying prospect for me.

I believe that there are many parallels between the "control" aspects of eating disorders and obsessive exercise routines. An awareness of these parallels and a willingness to keep them in check, as far as is possible, makes them, for me, manageable, if not always desirable.

It was not possible to exercise regularly during the last 10 weeks of my husband's life and there was a very noticeable, negative impact on my own physical and mental health as a consequence.

Since my husband died, and my life is no longer

dominated by endless rounds of hospital appointments, treatment sessions, consultations, blood tests, scans, etc, what had become an unhealthy obsession with completing my full exercise routine – regardless of whether or not I felt physically and/or emotionally able to do so – has settled back into a more healthy and enjoyable approach.

I still swim 6 mornings each week and walk several miles each day, but I now have a much more realistic attitude towards exercise once again. If I feel like doing my full swim, I do; if not, I don't!

As a result, I am enjoying my exercise routines again which is a much healthier, realistic, and sustainable way of living, getting fitter, and feeling better.

For me, there is nothing quite like the feeling of exhilaration at the end of every workout particularly so on those days when I don't want to be bothered. The benefits of structure, routine, shared exercise experience and endorphins are addictive, and I would encourage everyone to give them a try.... within your limitations, of course.

Chapter 12

Self-Protection: Change Fear into a SUPERPOWER

Jennie

When do most people stop and consider their security? I think to be honest it's an extremely low priority in most people's minds daily.

I hear so many comments such as

'I haven't been attacked yet.'

'I am ok, I know how to throw a punch.'

'Why would I need Self Defence skills? I don't want to become violent.'

It isn't an easy subject to discuss, but violence against women and girls is a reality within our society. Many women live in situations where they are bullied and coerced, that are potentially dangerous. and where they might face actual physical assault.

If this doesn't affect us, we can become oblivious to the problem, but in the UK alone, on average, four women a week are murdered by their partners. This is an appalling statistic, and yet is given very low publicity compared to, for example, the horrible but very rare incidents of people killed after being attacked by dangerous dogs.

It is true, of course, that **assault by strangers is extremely rare, a**nd it's not something most people think about.

Self Defence training is NOT just about our physical ability to protect ourselves, (that's another book in itself) but being able to protect ourselves from any sensation of fear we may experience.

Let's start by looking at what we can do daily to help keep ourselves safe. First, we need to understand fear.

Fear is a focused feeling of anxiety which is naturally triggered when we feel under threat. This is a very basic response common to all animals. Like the ability to feel pain, we possess it for a reason. It is there to keep us from harm.

Fear is a natural and adaptive emotion response to a perceived threat. It's perceived when we become aware or conscious of a threat. If we could look at fear as a form of energy we can understand and channel it more effectively.

Fear can manifest itself as a physiological response such an increase in our heart rate, adrenaline rush, and heightened alertness. This energy is the body's natural reaction to perceived threats or danger, preparing it to either confront or flee from the threat.

However, the energy from fear can also be mental and emotional, influencing our thoughts, behaviour and decision making. Sometimes fear is misplaced or can get out of hand.

When we learn how to manage our fears, we can channel our fear energy into the production of action for self-protection.

We human beings are complicated, and many people experience fear when it is not physically justified, but through social interactions. Social and mental perceived threats can trigger a response, when we experience the same sensations in the body as though we were in physical danger. Here are some examples of how fear can appear:

- Phobia
- Social Anxiety
- Fear of failure
- Fear of rejection
- Fear of uncertainty
- Existential fear
- Fear of loss
- Fear of the future
- Fear of pain or injury
- Existential Fear

We can see that these are like the general sensations of anxiety described in the previous chapter, and the recommended methods of dealing with general anxiety also apply to fears.

Fear can prevent us from doing and achieving many things, for example stepping into a gym for the first time. For someone this can be a massive fear, the fear of looking stupid, of not knowing what to do in the gym, the social fear of comparing ourselves to others.

Fear can steal our self-control, our ability to be aware, our ability to react and respond under pressure, our natural 'fight or flight mechanism' we need to deal with actual threats of harm.

Facing and dealing with fear can be a slow and gradual process, so reach out to ask for help if you are struggling on your own. Time, patience and practice will help you learn to effectively manage your fears and live a more fulfilling life.

The ability to control your fears is your first step to improving your security. Fear can steal your ability to be aware. Awareness and alertness are key qualities needed for self-protection and avoiding danger.

We need to be always aware, but when our heart rate is raised due to a possible potential attack this can act as a massive distraction to our minds.

Fear can bring on

- A Faster Heart Beat
- Sweating
- Rapid breathing

However, we can then use that surge of energy, and turn it to our advantage. It's like our very own Superpower, and an extremely powerful ability to possess.

Just imagine being able to identify your fears, to address them and turn those feelings into a superpower. Well, you can!

When it comes to looking after our security, identifying our fears can have such an impact on the way people can read us, we can generally spot someone who is feeling nervous.

"People who look like good victims are good victims."

But also, fear can sometimes make people abrupt and short tempered, which then can cause the same body language or verbal language to come back to them. This then easily can escalate into something physical.

Remember we are responsible for our own personal security, and we must start by controlling our fears. Conflict of one sort or another will inevitably occur in our lives, but it doesn't need to turn ugly or physical. If we have a genuine disagreement, for example with someone, we can learn how to resolve it without hostility or hurting the other person either mentally or physically.

This is not something some people find easy. They don't deal well with conflict and misunderstand the difference between aggression and assertiveness.

Assertiveness is very different from aggression or domination and comes from having a strong sense of self and quiet confidence in your strength and integrity. If you are quietly assertive and stand your ground in an argument, then you can deal with bullies and people who threaten you much more effectively.

Dealing with bullying is a vital skill, which many girls and women are sadly having to learn more and more these days, but a strong mind in a strong body is a brilliant defence against being bullied.

Both men and women can become bullies, but resorting to violence is never a good idea. and one of the great strengths of martial arts training is that it teaches and channels its students' self-knowledge and self-control.

Your ability to improve your own personal security can just be the start of a very powerful journey. Once you address those fears, you unleash hidden power. Just think of the person we referred to before, who had a fear of stepping into the gym.

Imagine the person's potential that they could unlock by having the courage to step into the gym and start their gym programme, to meet new friends, and even inspire others to take the same positive steps they have.

That then leads us to be able to exercise and improve our well-being at a powerful pace, whether or not we go to the gym to train for a certain goal. Mine is working towards my next Dan Grade in Martial Arts, so this motivates me each day to work towards that goal.

My wider personal goal is to be as fit as possible and to aim to be as healthy as I can. As I age, I find this harder to maintain, especially at the age of 48 when the hormones like to throw curve balls our way.

If anything, growing older makes me more determined as I want to keep my bone density, be able to carry heavy shopping bags, and be able to breathe easily.

This means that when it comes to self-defense, I believe our training starts with our well-being. We need to be able to be fit if we are to fight our challenges. These could be mental or physical challenges, health issues, or anything that life throws in our path.

By fighting I mean the ability to fight anything that life throws our way. If we are fit and alert and have learned to control our fears and channel them into positive energy, then we can overcome all the challenges that might face us.

Jennie's Own Story

My name is Jennie I am 48 years old this year, I am a mother to Gracie who is 18 years old, and a wife to my husband Stephen, and my favourite pastime is learning about Self-protection, mentally and physically. Some may say It's a strange hobby for a female, as generally self-protection training normally attracts males, and it's a male-dominated activity.

When I left school at 16 I didn't have a plan for my life, but that is me. I was already working at my Grandad's family business which was a garage and fuel station. I spent hours there working or generally being a nuisance to my dad.

So, at 16 when working at my grandfather's garage a local dentist came in

---

whom I knew. He asked me the good old question we ask all teenagers "So what are you going to do now, what do you want to do with your life?"

My reply was "Not really sure."

He said "I am looking for a dental nurse. You can start on Monday."

Monday arrived and there I was, standing in a dental surgeon clinic watching teeth getting filled or extracted, and guess what, I absolutely loved it! I qualified as a dental nurse in 1994 and I worked there until 2012 when my daughter Gracie was born.

After Gracie was born I then had a change of career and went into hairdressing and beauty and worked at my mum's salon with my sister for a few years. Thirteen years later, we closed the salon. My Mum was diagnosed with breast cancer, but she put up a strong fight and she is now in remission.

In school, sports were not my thing at all. Actually, I hated PE, but then I found Boxing, then progressed into Kickboxing, and then truly found what I was looking for was training for a purpose such as learning Self-protection.

Over my many years of training and learning about self-protection, I've seen many practices and training which is not helpful and even dangerous. But I truly believe, and know now that where I currently am with my training, I am training alongside the elite of Self-protection and feel confident sharing my experience and knowledge with others.

I achieved my first belt in 2019 and my second Dan black belt in 2020. I am now working towards gaining my third. There aren't too many female black belts compared to male black belts, I want to change that, hence why I became an instructor.

Training in Self-protection has very many benefits. It is not just about having the physical ability when it comes to being able to use your own body as your weapon of defence, but also educating yourself on how to keep your body (the most powerful weapon) fit to fight, fit to fight diseases too.

As you can imagine I have been training for many years and I am still training, still learning brand new skills, adapting my training to my life. Now it's all about battling the menopause and being determined that won't stop me.

I hear so many people blame things such as menopause for preventing them from training, but I would disagree. Once you have your mindset focused on why you are doing something, it will help you achieve your goals/ So don't make weight loss your only reason to go to the gym.

I am extremely lucky that I get to work and help people every day, I have some amazing people around me.

Chapter 13

Recovering From Addiction

Jennie and Susanne

What is addiction? It is anything that we have to do, that we can't give up, that rules our lives, and depletes our money. It turns us into its slaves.

It can ruin relationships, destroy the happiest of families, blight the lives of children and adults, and cause us to commit crimes and even cause death. Addiction to alcohol, tobacco, drugs like cocaine, cannabis or other narcotics, glue sniffing, and other physical addictions are obvious to an outsider because they affect our bodies and make us very ill.

The things that should nourish our minds and bodies become poison to us. Over-eating is classic addictive behavior. Even compulsive over-exercising and obsession with our body image can easily become an addiction.

But other, more hidden, addictions are just as powerful, like gambling, hoarding, or compulsive shopping. This is true across all social classes. Being rich doesn't protect you from becoming addicted.

Indeed, it sometimes promotes the problem.

The only benefit to having a large income is that it prevents you from being sent to jail for crimes you commit, to pay for your 'habit'. This is a very poor word to use in connection with addiction. One can usually break a habit, but if you suffer from a true addiction, then giving up can become incredibly painful. It becomes not a habit but a slave-master.

So how can we quit those 'bad habits' and develop new, good ones?

Overcoming addiction can be a long and hard process, but it is possible, as many people will testify. Katie's story, which she has shared below, is very powerful and honest, and it highlights the challenges of overcoming addiction.

The following pointers might help you take that first vital step toward recovery and eventual freedom. They are all equally important and may be the difference between disappointing failure and triumph.

1. **Take the First step**. Decide to quit: Your recovery starts with you choosing the future you want for yourself. Know you have the power to change your life, so commit to recovery. Focus on the great way you will feel once you have beaten the addiction. Think of the health benefits. Visualise your new self. Do this every

morning, and build affirming mantras into your daily routine.

2. **Prepare for the day when you will quit** and set things up so you have support, and the minimum of temptation. A day within the next two weeks is the best time, so you will not lose momentum. Treat it as a red-letter day on your calendar. It might be the most important date in the rest of your life.

3. **Enrol positive family members and friends.** Tell them what you want to do, and make them see how serious you are. But don't listen to anyone who encourages you to keep up your bad habits, or dismisses how important quitting is to you. This is very important, as we are so easily discouraged.

4. Changing one's fundamental mindset about an addiction, whatever it is, drugs, smoking, drinking, excess food, gambling etc. is much harder when people do not support you. Addicted people tend to hide away from others, who might confront them with awkward truths about what they are doing to themselves. This is the opposite of what you need to do.

5. **Get professional help** and join a support group if possible. Alcoholics Anonymous is still one of the most effective sources of support, friendship and advice in the world and has branches

everywhere. If you know you won't be able to quit by yourself, go to see your doctor and explain. They will refer you to a counsellor or therapist who specialises in curing addiction, or refer you to a support group. Doctors will do this willingly as they want to see you in good health.

6. **Change your routine**. Avoid going to places where you have indulged your addiction in the past. It might be restaurants or pubs, bars, or the local betting shop. If you are a gambler, take the bookmakers' apps off your phone, and avoid watching the sporting activities on TV that fuelled your addiction in the past.

7. **Prepare for when you relapse** as this is normal, especially after the first one or two weeks, as the addiction fights to stay in your body. But don't panic, if it happens, just start again. Remove temptation by of course taking out of the house and destroying any supplies of whatever it is you are addicted to.

8. **Make sure you are otherwise in as good health** as you can achieve. Are you getting enough sleep, eating healthy foods, and exercising regularly? Katie's story shows just how helpful it was for her to work with a personal fitness trainer to improve her health, overcome her addiction and other mental health issues, and achieve great physical fitness, despite having

suffered so much pain and illness after a bad accident.

Reflection by Katy: Recovering from Addiction.

*Even though I am only in my mid-twenties, I have struggled with my **physical and mental health for some time now.** I have struggled with pain and mobility problems after a camel accident while I was on holiday in Egypt. The pain made work life difficult when I returned home, physically, and mentally, and I eventually started using cocaine and other substances as a coping mechanism.*

Then I developed an eating disorder and stopped eating and drinking. I became addicted to cocaine as it seemed to give me lots of energy which I needed, as I felt so tired from my prescription medication and not eating or drinking. It lifted my mood as I was suffering from mental health problems, and it helped me continue to work.

I lost a lot of weight and at my worst I was only 7 stone. But I started using more and more cocaine as I found that the effects were not lasting as long. I lost all my savings, thousands of pounds, and before long I became very ill. I had to give up my job as I could no longer cope. This made my mental health worse as I lost my whole routine, social life and purpose.

The turning point came when my parents discovered that I was using cocaine and were very worried and upset. They were very supportive and made me promise to stop before I died.
I had overdosed several times before they found out but I didn't tell them as that would have upset them even more. I decided to listen to my parents and accepted their help to start recovery as I knew if I carried on I would soon die.

For the first few months I felt exhausted like I had no energy and this made the cravings very difficult as I felt as though I needed the Cocaine to fuel my body. My nose was very painful from snorting Cocaine. I couldn't imagine life without Cocaine. I felt hopeless but stuck to my promise to my parents.

We started off cutting down slowly and they gave me a date that would be my last day of using Cocaine. That day was 17th July 2020.

My mum helped distract me from my cravings by playing games with me and getting me out of the house. We celebrated every milestone in secret and it slowly got easier to cope without it. But I wasn't out of the woods yet. I became more and more ill due to my eating disorder and was admitted to hospital, malnourished and dehydrated. Because of my mental state and being unable to eat I was sectioned and fitted with a feeding tube.

I was in hospital for six months, and spending this amount of time in hospital stuck in bed caused my muscles to waste and become weak. I struggled to walk and had lots of falls and had to use a wheelchair. After leaving hospital I decided to join the gym to build myself back up.

There I met my personal trainer and she began helping me to get stronger and more mobile. She planned our sessions at a pace I could cope with and concentrated on building up my strength and improving my mobility. She also helped me to start eating again by suggesting different foods to try and helping me plan and cook my meals.

My mental health started to improve. I started to feel better and better and became more mobile. My energy levels started to increase. I started being able to walk independently without the use of a wheelchair.

I never thought I could feel so good about myself without cocaine but now I feel so much better than cocaine ever made me feel. I work out every day now and my physical and mental health are great. I still take medication for pain in my back and legs from the accident and medication for my mental health.

I feel stable now and very fit. I am happy with my life and really enjoy my fitness training. My personal trainer is supporting me and is always there to give me helpful advice on exercise and nutrition. I have recently had my feeding tube removed. It has been three years now since I quit Cocaine and took back control of my life.

Katie Bellamy

Chapter 14

Time – The most precious thing in the world.

Susanne

One of the most frequent excuses I hear from people is that they can't get fit, because they simply don't have the time to go to the gym. They feel like the white rabbit in the Victorian classic children's book, *Alice in Wonderland,* who rushes past Alice, complaining he has to run, and can't stop to talk, he has no time for anything! Aren't we so often like that poor white rabbit, rushing from pillar to post, trying to cram too many things into a day, and juggling all our competing responsibilities?

Men and women have different attitudes towards time, in my experience. I think, for so many women, we see time as a threatening thing in its scarcity. There is never enough time for all our many conflicting responsibilities and all the things we must achieve in a day. There just doesn't seem any time to do what we want to do, and when we do take an hour for ourselves, we can be so full of guilt that we're wasting time, that we can't settle into it. I don't know many men who feel like this.

Now I'm retired from full-time work, my life is much less time-poor, but in my career as an international project assessor, I was always working to deadlines, made worse by knowing that people's lives might depend on my making the right decision, and even more importantly, on getting my reports written and submitted on time.

I know I felt like this for a long time and now until I learned to plan my life and manage my time, I perpetually felt guilty. I was wrong, and while it's taken me a while to learn, I know now that an hour spent alone, in sorting out my priorities for the day ahead or thinking through the best way to solve any problems that come up is my most valuable use of time.

I also know that if I don't spend at least an hour a day caring for my fitness, I will pay for it with sleepless nights, aching muscles, and a general feeling of malaise. What a waste of time that will be.

In the past, I wasted too much time very largely in fretting and worrying and this is something that I think I share with so many other people, even though by nature I am not a natural worrier. Think of it like this:

Researchers have said that about 50% of the time we worry about things that will never happen, and 30% of the time we worry over decisions we made in the past we cannot alter. Then 12% of our worrying time is taken up with health concerns which may come to nothing, and which we can't reasonably do much about and so out of 100% of all the worrying we do, only 8% is taken up with genuine problems. Half of those things we have no control over anyway, so we really should only worry about 4% of the things that might come our way. So, what a waste of time all that time worrying is!

In writing about the importance of planning and good timekeeping, the first thing I would say try to stop worrying! It's such an energy-sapping, depressing activity.

Someone once said to me "Are you a plate spinner or a plate smasher? In writing terms, a common question is "Are you a plotter or a 'pantser'?"

Women very often try to try to be both. We want to be organised, but very often we run along managing our lives by the seat of our pants. We become a frantic plate spinner as we juggle responsibilities without prioritising them.

What are your plates? Many of us must juggle home life and work life. Our responsibilities may also be to our elderly parents, children, spouses, and even to our pets. We feel guilty if we ever say no to anything.

We juggle all these things and in doing so we are bound to drop some things and very often the things we drop are the things that end up being the most important. Some things, like time to listen to loved ones, or to feed our imagination, once lost have been lost forever.

So, the big question is what can we do to make more time, make more time, for fun, physical exercise, for listening and for being still? To make more time to extend our life we need to become fit and in doing so we could extend our life by up to a decade!

Just think, time, like soil, and water is finite. It is infinitely precious, so there's no point wasting it in trivial things that don't matter. We might miss the wood for the trees if we put too great an emphasis on how we look, how our house looks, how clean the car is, even how well-behaved our children are.

Imagine if everything was to be taken away from us, as has happened so tragically in many places in the world this year when we're left with nothing as our house has been blown up or lost in a flood, our lands have dried up under climate change and we have no food to feed our babies, so we have to leave, carrying all our possessions on our backs. Can you imagine how that will make us prioritise in a very different way?

I'm not saying that everybody, or even anybody, reading this book will have to face those dreadful decisions, but life does throw a wobbly now and then. I take comfort in the fact that if I suddenly lose my life, I have planned sufficiently so I will be able to leave my basic affairs in good order for my loved ones and family.

Now this may not be so applicable to many people under my age. (72.) But we are all faced with big decisions on how we order our lives, at any stage.

For example, if you're young you might want to talk about planning to start a family or take out a mortgage on your own house. There's been a lot of talk recently about couples even putting off having children because of the pressures on daily budgets.

Now, I would like to talk more straightforwardly about planning day by day, week by week, and month by month. Every journey needs a destination, but we also need to know how to get there. I'm amused very often by the fact that many younger people have no idea where places are in the country because they rely on Satnav.

You type in the address where you want to go and

a satellite in the sky far above your head will automatically and very politely take you there. I had a friend who took his family on holiday all the way from Yorkshire to the Isle of Wight but afterwards he couldn't say where he'd been, whether it was north or south even, because the Satnav did all the decision-making for him!

Sometimes the whole of our lives can feel like that. We let others, or passing fashions we see on the internet, decide for us. I think it's not a bad idea to go back to the old idea of having a map. This isn't just a geographical map, but a life map that sets out where you want to go and provides you with more than some vague idea about how to get there.

If I say I want to lose 20 lbs, and I want to get much stronger muscles, so I'll be able to lift my grandchildren and run up and down stairs in a few years, I need to plan the way to get there. I don't have an electronic Satnav for life, that I can just plug into. Despite all the gadgets, like smartwatches and Fitbits, I must do a little bit of work myself planning how I'm going to achieve my dreams.

I'm a great believer in having a wall chart so that you can see visually what things are happening throughout the year ahead. Also, if you have long-term projects like mine, you need a long-term perspective.

Because I write books, I always have to plan up to six months ahead to know when I can get in the writing time, when I can put in the space to get the book edited and formatted, and then to have it proofread and reviewed. If I don't do this then there's no way that the book will ever see the light of day.

Good planning brings freedom and can guarantee enhanced achievement. For a few years a long time ago, I taught A-level students Politics and History and some of my students very often came into class on a Monday morning unfit to learn anything. They'd been out drinking and carousing over the weekend and were badly hung over.

I used to say. "Realign your behaviour and attitude to your goals. Remind yourselves of your hopes for the future, and then compare them with what you're doing or not doing in practice to achieve them." (Teachers sometimes do talk like this!)

I needed to give them a reality check and recenter their position on the road to their hopes and dreams.

I invented one little formula that said for every grade they hoped to achieve at A level they needed to put in at least 50 hours of personal study. If the students wanted to get an A grade that meant they should study for 200 hours on top of classroom-based assignments for each subject.

Now studying 200 hours over the space of two years was very achievable, even though the idea at first shocked my poor students! But by breaking down the work that they must put in, into manageable chunks, and sticking to the plan, they did achieve their aims and goals.

In terms of fitness, this is even more achievable and a very sensible way forward. There are many apps. available these days which claim to help us do various workouts and how to increase our level of fitness. Most of them cost money to join and people so often start well, and then fall by the wayside. It's a waste of time and money to do this, so take your planning into your own hands.

At the beginning of every month, I have a clear-out session of my working space, on and off-line. First, I balance my budget for the previous month and make sure all bills are paid. Then I clear out any papers still lying in the in-tray.

Some people never leave their workstation each day, unless all papers are dealt with, and it's a wonderful rule if you can hold each piece of paper only once. The idea that a messy and overcrowded desk or worktop indicates a creative and brilliant mind is nonsense.

We haven't got time here to talk in-depth about the problem of procrastination, but it is an interesting psychological factor that procrastinators are usually very highly stressed, good people, riddled with guilt about not achieving what they want to achieve. They punish themselves by delaying even longer.

It is a sign of anxiety when you put off very basic things, not necessarily expensive activities or things that would take up a huge amount of time. You cause mental 'self-harm' by overloading your abilities to cope with stress, and of course, tomorrow will be even more painful.

There's been a lot written recently about the psychology of procrastination and it is very interesting, but for now, all I would say is why not create a daily list of what you hope to achieve and divide it into three short sections, the things you have to do to make life easy for others, the things that you need to do to make life easy for yourself, and the things that you'd like to do and then get on and do them! The sense of freedom you will feel will be wonderful.

Having arranged a monthly chart of planned activities, make sure that once a week you do take a rest day from what you normally must do in a week. People may say, "I'm working an eight-hour day already. Then I have all the housework to do at the weekend. I've no time for any time off."

A full-time job still leaves 16 hours a day. It's a

matter of allowing yourself to take time out for yourself, permission many women find it impossible to give themselves. But if you have an ambition to become physically fitter, then you must make the necessary space in your life.

Virginia Woolf said that any woman who wanted to be a creative writer had to have a room of their own. I would add that any woman who wants to become fighting fit must have at least one hour a day in which she can have a total choice in how to spend her time.

One way of running my working day which works to my strengths as a freelance writer, is to use the time-block system. I block the day off in 2-hour sections and work my schedule around these.

I know my best energies and powers of concentration are focused in the morning. I'm a lark, rather than an owl, and so I can get up at 4, 5 or 6:00 a.m. if I need to, to complete a project. I love writing in the early dawn and open my windows to hear the birdsong in the dawn chorus as I open my computer and start the day's work.

But ask me to do the same sort of work at 4, 5, or 6:00 in the afternoon, and then I will be far less efficient and far less focused. I will be weary, so that's not a good time of day for me to put in a lot of intellectual 'brain' work.

I find going to the gym a very good way of recovering after an early writing two-hour time block, so I like to visit the gym around 8 am. where I can get some exercise, swim, run, or do a short half-hour workout. There I can then take a hot shower and sort out my hair, makeup, and clothes for the rest of the day before joining friends for a chat in the reception lounge over the morning papers and perhaps a decaf. coffee.

Because I follow an intermittent fasting regime, this works for me, because I then return home for a light breakfast around 10:00. I then work again at the desk until midday when I begin to prepare lunch from scratch, usually something light.

My husband and I eat our main meal together at about 1:00 pm while watching the midday news, and in the afternoon, I prefer to work outside in the garden when the weather allows or take a walk perhaps with our dog. If I try to work longer than two hours at the desk in one session my focus tends to wander and I'm less efficient.

It's never good to sit for a long time in one position, so I regularly jump up and move about for a mad five minutes. There's also plenty of time after lunch, to go shopping or socialise, and to do the necessary housework. (My husband cleans the house while I take care of the laundry.)

I've retired from paid employment, so this pattern of life is easy for me, but I know many people who are still employed, yet still manage to find time for themselves within a very busy working week. I'm sure the best way to cope is to always have one hour of quiet reflection every day in which you stop fretting, and do something that absorbs you.

For some, this might be at the gym doing a very physical activity, or you might choose simply to sit in a quiet room, with all the electronics turned off.

There you can close your eyes and take a ten-minute meditation. Even this amount of time-out will refresh your brain and help you cope with the demands of the day.

I am a great believer in accountability and sticking to a regular commitment. This is how slimming clubs work, as they don't leave you alone to backslide for more than a week. They ask you to return at the same time every week to weigh in, to be accountable for what you've done, and to listen to words of encouragement from other people, so it keeps you on track.

Getting into a good new habit means doing it daily for at least three weeks, and then sticking at it for the long run. If you want to lose ten or twenty pounds, it's no good just having one salad and then thinking you've cracked the problem. You need to start eating salads every day!

Having a salad must become a daily habit. It's much more positive to start a new, good habit, than to feel life is all about having to give up bad habits, which is much harder.

But what happens if you hit a roadblock and the goal you are pursuing becomes unattainable? Some natural human problems or disasters are bound to happen at times. You, or your partner might lose your job, meaning you may have to make massive re-adjustments. Illness or an accident may intervene.

Don't despair and don't give up. Like the satnav does in the car, simply 'adjust your route plan'. These things are all part of normal life, but if you have a commonsense, balanced approach to life and plan on a weekly basis, you can still succeed.

President Barack Obama was asked what his secret power was. How was he able to be the president of the USA and stay so calm under all that stress and provocation?

He answered that he didn't think he had special powers, but he did one thing which always gave him an advantage. He made sure he was always early for every meeting or activity. He never ran late.

This meant he could get to a meeting ten minutes before it started, and so was prepared in his mind and paperwork to cope with what might be thrown at him. By doing this one small thing, he gave himself a superpower.

It's as easy to be ten minutes early as it is to be ten minutes late. Think about it. You only need to do it once, and your whole life can readjust thereafter.

I liked that idea and I've tried to work with it. Now I find being late is discourteous to others, and usually avoidable. Though of course, I can still fall and turn up late, as we all can.

For example, I know that if I must drive through a busy town, it's best to allow an extra 30 minutes at certain times of day. Once a week I drive twelve miles to pick up my grandchildren from school and give them tea.

If I leave home too late, I will hit all the school traffic going into their town, but if I leave early then everything will be smooth and I will be in good time, waiting at the school gate for their cheery faces to emerge. Simple adjustments like that can improve one's whole day, with just a little bit of planning.

The other thing that people often find very stressful, is when our household machinery and gadgets don't work well and we don't think outside the box enough for solutions. I read of somebody who complained that her dishwasher never really made things clean, and this upset and annoyed her. It happened regularly, and meant that she always, very grumpily, had to take everything out of the machine and re-wash the crockery and cutlery by hand.

This went on, until one day a friend said to her, "Why don't you simply run the dishwasher a second time? No-one is telling you that you can't." This suggestion transformed her experience and changed how she thought about everything else she did. She didn't need permission to improve her life.

There's always an easy way to achieve efficiency in daily chores, for example how to pull out a drawer that sticks. We can ease the drawer runners by putting on some WD40 or rubbing candle wax, or a bar of soap along them and never have to push and shove again.

We can also make our lives very much easier if we apply some metaphorical WD40 or oil to whatever we do. By planning and arranging our time according to our strengths, we can make our time stretch to accommodate all the things we need and would like to do. I still believe time is the most precious gift we are given, and knowing how to use it well can transform our life for the better!

Chapter 15

The last two decades - Facing the future with confidence, whatever your age!

Susanne

If every moment of our lives is a precious irreplaceable thing, then the last decades of our lives on earth are as important as any other time. Do you remember the song from the musical "Gypsy"? Who wants to spend life sitting in a sitting room? Let's live life right to the end, not just sitting or residing in retirement, but running at full tilt until we collapse in a heap by the roadside like an old bicycle. Wouldn't that be more fun?

There are so many wrongs to be righted in the world, so many people who need help, so many lonely souls who could do with a friend. You can feel old at fifty and young at ninety, but if you are fit, strong and vigorous, it's your duty to enjoy that gift, not turn your back on new ideas, and just sit down with your feet up.

I've never really been impressed with the idea of

retirement, with all that it means in terms of not doing what you want to do, not still stretching yourself, and not enjoying life to the full. The idea of downsizing to a very small bungalow, where you have no room to turn around, of coping on a small income and becoming a 'pensioner', all conjure up ideas of loss, restriction, and the assumption that there's nothing much to look forward to.

In my mind, nothing could be further from the truth of reaching the final decades, and not only do we need to reexamine those last ten or twenty years of our life, but we also might think about death as the next great adventure, a door into a new creative and unknown state of being.

There's nothing gruesome about this; it's the one truth about life. The one sure thing we know about our creator is that we are born fresh and equipped with all we need to lead a great life, but that even after 100 years our time on earth will finish in our death.

For many young people, even talking about arranging a funeral or where we'd like to be buried seems scary. However, the older we are, the more philosophical we become, and I think planning for death needs to be taken seriously. A well-planned death can be one of the most sensible gifts we can leave our loved ones.

Both of my parents lived into their 90th years and

I have one great, great grandfather who was a professional gardener, who lived from before the Battle of Waterloo until the start of World War One, so I probably have a fighting chance of becoming a feisty old lady.

I'd quite like to turn into what was called in medieval times a *crone*. I like that word, which is a good way of describing a woman who is wise, knowledgeable, and strong, and who takes no nonsense from anybody. When you're an old crone you should rattle your sticks at fate and battle on.

A week or so before he died, I was visiting my ninety-seven-year-old father-in-law as he lay on what was to become his deathbed, when he said to me, "I need to go! It's time to go!"

"Of course, Dad," I said soothingly. "You've had a good life, just accept what comes next and relax into it."

"No, no," he said. "I need to go! Fetch the nurse and ask for a bedpan!" No, he didn't intend to depart quietly at all.

None of us can know what's going to happen after our death. We may have faith that there's an afterlife, or we may assume that our carbon atoms simply return to the earth from which we came.

But we're not there yet. How best to face the

challenge of our seventies, eighties, or nineties? How can we keep creating new memories?

Of course, old age brings with it many challenges, as someone famous (I can't remember who!) said, old age is not for wimps. For starters, it generally brings bereavement with it. With great love comes great pain with its loss, and to be bereaved in a loving partnership is a raw and painful business.

Physical challenges, with hearing, eyesight, or memory loss, can if we let them, depress us and hold us back. Many people are in constant pain in old age, which is a horrible thing to have to deal with. It saps our energy, takes away our self-confidence, and often makes us depressed. As many as one in four people endure severe long-term pain, and it is not understood or given enough resources within the current medical climate.

But there is still so much we can do, and I am sure the answer is to be ready to adapt and adjust, and not cling to a previous way of life, or to possessions that no longer serve us in the way they perhaps did once.

So, how do you approach the challenge of staying fighting fit, once you're well past 70 and into your 80s or even 90s?

I have many older friends who inspire and amuse me, and sometimes irritate me. That's how it should be. They always stimulate me by the intense life force I feel still emerges from them.

Keeping good friends is vital to avoiding loneliness and stagnation. You might also make new friends, unexpectedly by joining a church, a gym, or a social group, like a book group for example, or why not join a running club and start training for a half marathon? (I'm not joking!)

I have one housebound friend who writes weekly letters, not of complaint, but of encouragement to people she approves of, often to politicians or campaigners who normally get hate mail. One word of praise is worth a hundred of criticism. (Now that stamps cost so much though, she has taken to emailing her messages more often than posting them.)

One of the best ways of staying young and having a youthful outlook is to expect to make new friends. Sometimes, in old age, people retreat into themselves and don't feel they have the energy to make new connections or to take an interest in what's happening around them. But closeness to young people, like our own grandchildren, if we are lucky enough to have them, or perhaps the children at a nearby primary school can be a great thing, and very positive.

Volunteers to hear children read are usually welcomed with open arms in all schools. Chatting to five or seven-year-olds will soon liven you up. Acting your age, and sticking just in the company of your contemporaries, isn't always the best way to carry on.

On the other hand, why is there such a cult now among women past the menopause of trying to look twenty years younger? Any women can pretend they have long thick blonde hair and large breasts like nursing mothers. But isn't it rather silly to pretend to still be fertile, when we're not?

What is interesting is that human females are the only animals whose life span far outlasts their breeding capacity. Obviously, we are very much still needed in the tribe. There is no need to pretend we are still going to procreate after the age of fifty.

So, are there special attributes of old age we need to examine and do something about? Of course. One thing is bone loss through osteoporosis. This is something I'm conscious of, for my mother lost seven inches in height to the condition through her eighties, and eventually, I could look down at her. The pain of fragile bones and possible fractures can be life changing and makes us scared of falling over.

Supplements of calcium, coupled with eating lots of dark green vegetables, and plenty of protein are essential for bone health. But weight-bearing exercises can have a major effect as well. Weightlifting for older women is an excellent exercise to start, however old you are, as is any consistent programme of exercise, even if you are chair-bound.

One way in which people experiment now to regain youthful vim and vigour is to cut down on the calories in their diet quite substantially in old age. A well-balanced diet with good protein, fresh vegetables and strong mineral and vitamin intake can sustain very good health, even if you reduce it to around 1300 calories a day. In some research projects, this has been found to increase lifespan by forty percent. (Of course, most of this research was done on mice!)

I'm a strong believer in a diet consisting of mostly fresh, organic vegetables, and while I still eat meat and sustainably caught fish, I'm turning more and more towards an organic plant-based diet. For me, this will include eggs of course, because my husband produces the best free-range organically produced eggs that I've ever seen. We sell them at the gate with the tag: *Garnett's Garden Eggs, laid while you wait.*

A recent series on Netflix has examined the lifestyle of six of the oldest populations in the world and found they share similar attributes. These ninety-year-olds are largely vegetarian, eat loads of yoghurt, nuts, and sweet potatoes, have a strong sense of community and mutuality, and they keep working and walking up and down steep hills. Retirement is a word they rarely use, but they play a full and vital role within their extended families and in their neighborhoods.

In the absence of close family, keeping an animal like a dog or a cat is the next best thing for happiness in old age. Some people say that animals are preferable to humans, as they give so much love and approval and provide us with those much-needed hugs we mentioned earlier. Also taking the dog for a walk keeps the nation fitter than almost any other activity. In times of extreme grief, knowing you have a little dog or cat depending on you to feed and care for it, can make all the difference to whether you want to carry on living.

There was an interview recently on the television with Joan Collins, who provides an extreme example of defying old age with a certain pizzazz. But we have many excellent examples in other famous actors, like Dame Judy Dench, or Dame Maggie Smith, who show no desire to retire in their late eighties and nineties.

We don't need to be celebrities to follow the same attitude. In our own lives, we will know our role models. So, let's run forward into the last decades of our life expecting fun and frolics, and who knows, even fresh love and romantic adventures!

Anne's testimony

Since the age of 70, my life has taken a very different direction to earlier years, and I am amazed at the wide range of activities with which I have been involved. One thing seems to have led to another.

Around twelve months after my husband of 48 years died, I felt I wanted to widen my range of activities beyond the varied church responsibilities that I had undertaken for many years.

The first was to be involved in a voluntary capacity as a member of Student Support Services at my local university. This brought me a new perspective on the challenges that meet the modern-day student.

From my work there I learned of an opportunity to volunteer overseas, and off I went to Sri Lanka for three months to work in the Theological College. This led to me being accepted as a Mission Partner of the Methodist Church. So, at 76, I undertook paid employment, a two-year placement back in Sri Lanka.

Challenges abounded, if I had both water and electricity for my morning shower it was a good day but rice three times a day was rather too much. There was great joy in living with mainly young people, enthusiastic about their learning.

I have returned to Sri Lanka a couple of times since to meet up with friends, meet former students now involved in their careers, and to visit projects in remote areas of the island.

Since COVID-19, I have undertaken mentoring folk who are exploring their vocations in the Methodist Church. Zoom is a great asset here!

I continue to look forward to new challenges. My mantra is "All I have is now". I do enjoy having friends of a wide age range, several different interest groups, and gently exercising most days of the week. The pleasure of splashing around and swimming at my local leisure club comes from the relief it gives from painful joints. I have arthritis and the swimming pool is the only place where I am pain-free! I also attend an age-appropriate exercise class once a week.

Now I am eighty-two I have accepted that there are some things I have had to let go, which is not always an easy thing to do, but I find fresh opportunities come along! I am about to leave for another three-week visit to Sri Lanka, to meet my dear friends there and see where I may be of use again.

Anne Baldwin

February 2024

Chapter 16

Opening the door to the future. Where do you want to go from here?

Jennie and Susanne

We said at the beginning of the book that this is an introduction to a new way of life in which feeling fighting fit will be the normal way you'll feel in the future. There are some simple steps to achieve this, but there are no miracle methods, and no shortcuts. It will take some months, but it needn't take longer than that before you see and feel the difference.

We've learned about the complexities of the human body and the wonderful interaction of our mind, nervous system, our skeleton, organs, and muscles. The human body is a beautiful and exciting organism designed to do the best job of keeping us fit and healthy.

Everything is interconnected, and the small pituitary gland at the base of our brain almost magically keeps everything functioning through the performance of our various hormones.

All we have to do is treat our bodies well and kindly and gently discipline them in the best way forward. As we draw to the conclusion of this book, we'd like to encourage you to take some simple steps to reach your goals.

1. Know yourself, and love yourself too!

If you have managed to stay the course you all have learned that first of all it's important to know yourself inside and out and sometimes that can be a challenge. Having done it, then make sure your body knows you love it, that it is special and unique, and your best friend. Stop criticising it!

2. Start with a dream.

Dream of how you would like to be in 12 months. Visualise that dream. Make it real, then bring it into your mind as often as you can. Think how you are going to feel when you are fighting fit, and what you will be able to achieve. Imagine how good you're going to feel.

3. Kick out Mr Negativity.

We've spent quite a lot of time in the book talking about mental health and happiness and how to overcome anxiety so having visualised your dream, The next thing to do is to turn on happy thoughts and push away the voice of negativity and discouragement. They may come from other people. They may come from your circumstances but mostly they probably come from inside your head. So just say No to those thoughts and Yes to the new strong person that you can become.

4   **Be practical.** Make a time plan to reach your goals. Having got yourself into the right frame of mind the next thing to do is to make a series plan to look at how fitness and a new healthier way of eating can fit into the timetable of your life, and make sure that there is at least an hour a day that is just for you.

5   **Get outside!** If you work largely indoors, looking at a computer all day, make sure at least part of this hour is spent outside in the fresh air. We all need vitamin D so we all need sunshine and if we can't get that we will become depressed. Kickstart your new life by going outside and enjoying the fresh air whatever the season, whatever the time of year.

6.   **Move the body**. Ideally every day, but at least three times a week you need to start building movement into your life. Any movement is

good but movement which raises your heart level a little way above its normal resting rate will help improve your health and general fitness.

7. **Find a gym and a personal trainer**. The next thing we would advise you to do is to find your nearest or most accessible gym or fitness centre. Every town will have at least one, and you can always compare them by visiting more than one. Don't be scared! Listen to what your friends or neighbours recommend, and compare prices and the facilities on offer. Most gyms should offer a complimentary first visit, and a chance to discuss your needs with a personal trainer.

   Look for a sympathetic personal trainer and decide on your options. Don't spend more than you can afford. Even a single session can set you up with a personal work out and give you the right guidelines to get you started.

8. **Stay the Course.** Whether you may be able to commit to a single meeting with a trainer, a link-up once every two weeks, or a concentrated regime of a daily meeting over a short space of time, your trainer will give you a personal programme of exercises designed to take you from the place where you are now

slowly and surely to somewhere where you are feeling stronger fitter more energetic happier and more effective in meeting the challenges life will throw at you.

9. **Show up in Person.** There are so many online programmes giving exercise and diet ideas, but don't you think you need to meet your trainer? If you go to your local gym, they will assess you in person and give you a serious and professional service in finding the right exercises for you. Ask them anything you don't understand. They may show you around some frightening-looking machines that you may not even know how to use. But after a visit where the trainer will explain them to you, they will soon become very easy to manage and you can work slowly and surely until you can be stronger and lift, push, and pull much more than you can at the beginning.

10. **Think of food as fuel, delicious fuel.** But not your only friend. Do not continually top up your tank. Try to maintain a slight calorie deficiency. In terms of weight loss, if that is your aim, it is down to what and how much you eat which will determine how much weight you lose.

Physical exercise will make you fitter but your

diet will determine how many pounds you lose,
or, if you need to, how many pounds you gain,
because not everybody needs to lose weight.
Some of us are far too thin for our own good
and need more nutrition.

11. **Bye, Bye, Sugar!** Gently steer your mindset
away from the instant gratification of wanting
sweet things. Sugar is the most one of the most
addictive substances in the world today and
getting off it can be harder than giving up
smoking or even heroin. But you can do it.

12. **Think Long-term and Long distance**. One
thing we can guarantee, if you stick to a fitness
and eating healthily regime, you will see a
dramatic change in how you look and you will
also feel a dramatic change in how you feel
about yourself. But one swallow doesn't make
a summer. One salad won't make you skinny.
But stay committed and you will succeed.

**Finally, Good-bye and Good Luck. And look
forward to our next book, "How to Get Fighting
Fit."**

Appendix 1

Recipes for Success

Everybody likes a recipe. Here are some healthy ideas!

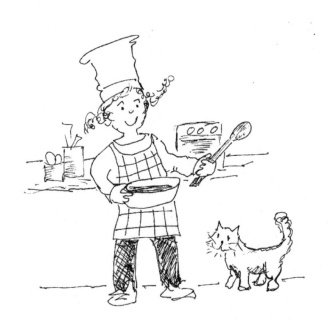

Herbivore Heaven Summer Pea Soup

Serves 4 to 6

Note: An American measuring cup is 8 oz, but you can use any cup as long as you stay consistent.

Ingredients:

- 3 tablespoons extra virgin olive oil
- 2 leeks, white and light green parts only, cleaned and sliced into circles.
- Salt to taste
- 4 cups frozen or fresh peas (1 ½ pounds – 2 12-oz bags frozen)
- 1 large iceberg lettuce, chopped.
- 5 cups chicken stock, vegetable stock or water
- ¼ cup coarsely chopped flat-leaf parsley leaves
- ¼ cup coarsely chopped fresh mint leaves
- ¼ cup chopped chives, plus additional for garnish
- Chopped fresh tarragon, chives and/or mint for garnish

Method:

1. Heat 1 tablespoon of the oil over medium heat in a large, heavy soup pot or Dutch oven, and add the leeks and a pinch of salt. Cook, stirring, until tender, about 5 minutes.

2. Add the peas, lettuce and stock or water, and bring to a boil. Add salt to taste. Reduce heat, cover, and simmer for 10 minutes or until the peas are tender. Remove from the heat and allow the vegetables and the broth to cool for 15 minutes. Taste the broth and season as desired.

3. Working in batches if necessary, blend the vegetables and herbs with the broth and additional olive oil for 2 minutes until smooth and the herbs have been absorbed. Return to the pot stir and reheat gently, or pour into a large bowl and continue to combine. Taste and adjust seasons.

4. If serving cold, chill for several hours. (This tastes wonderful cold.)

5. Serve, garnishing with a spoon of yogurt or crème fresh.

Pure and Simple Tomato Mousse starter

Serves 4

Ingredients:

- 6 ripe tomatoes
- Salt and pepper to taste

Method:

1. Skin 6 ripe tomatoes by dipping them in boiling water. The skin will easily slip off.
2. Blitz tomatoes in a food processor until fully combined.
3. Add a generous pinch of salt and pepper
4. Pour mixture into four small glasses
5. Place in the fridge overnight.

You will have four set mousse-like pots of deliciousness. No need for gelatine. The tomatoes will do their own thing.

Hot Weather Smoothie

Ingredients:

- 1/2 cup frozen Raspberries
- 1/2 cup frozen Blueberries
- 1 frozen Banana
- 3/4 – 1 cup Orange Juice

Method:

Whizz together in your blender or smoothie maker and serve. You can substitute frozen strawberries for the blueberries if you prefer a pinker look.!

Delicious.

Angelic Eggs

Ingredients:

- 6 large free-range eggs
- Light margarine
- Salt and pepper to taste
- 1 tsp English mustard
- 1 tsp paprika
- 1 tbsp sweet chili sauce

Method:

1. Hard boil six large free-range eggs and allow to cool (Note: Peeling is easier if they are not newly laid. Roll on a flat surface to loosen the shell and then remove the shells.
2. Halve each egg and remove yoks into a small bowl.
3. Add the margarine, salt, pepper, mustard, paprika and sweet chili sauce to the yolks and mash together well.
4. Pile the yolk mixture back into the whites.
5. Sprinkle with more paprika.
6. Serve chilled.

Main meals

Hot Weather Pastry

This works even when it's hot enough outside to fry an egg on the pavement. I was given this recipe in the Philippines. The pastry rolls out well and holds its shape. It is good for flans and quiches. Do not add any sugar.

Enough for two nine-inch pie crusts.

Ingredients:

- 3 cups of plain or self-rising flour. See previous recipe for note on the use of cups.
- 2/3 cup of milk
- 1/3 cup light vegetable oil
- Pinch Salt and pepper

Method:

1. Combine the oil and milk and then stir into the flour until it forms a ball of dough. Try not to use your hands too much.
2. Place in the fridge to chill for twenty minutes.
3. Roll out and use for pies and tarts.

4. You can now make up a healthy quiche by adding a mixture of 4 beaten eggs to 8oz grated cheese, and the cooked veg of your choice. Add steamed asparagus for luxury or grated carrots for a nice budget meal.

In winter, try this tasty Rootin', Tootin' Bean Stew

Serves four

Ingredients:

- 1 15oz Can of Borlotti, kidney or butter beans.
- 1 shallot (large)
- 1/2 leek
- two cloves of garlic. - chubby if not downright fat
- 1 large carrot
- 1/2 swede
- 1/2 large turnip
- 1 parsnip
- 2 potatoes
- a handful of savoy cabbage leaves, chopped.
- Marmite/Vegemite
- Worcestershire sauce
- Sweet chili sauce
- Sat and pepper
- Dried herbs
- Honey

Note: I used dried Borlotti beans from my garden, soaked overnight, but you can use any substantial can of beans, which makes the cooking process much quicker. For my stew, I used the following leftover vegetables in the fridge. You, of course, can make your own choice here. I am not your boss.

Method:

1. Peel and chop the veg, in different shapes and lengths but all roughly 2cms across.
2. Melt two tbsps. of vegetable oil in the pan and gently fry the vegetables until they soften slightly, adding them in turn as listed above, the onion and softer veggies first followed by the others.
3. Then add one tin of Borlotti, red kidney, or butter beans.
4. Fill the tin with vegetable stock, using a bouillon cube if you don't have fresh stock. and pour over the vegetables. Repeat.
5. I used up a good dollop of Marmite/Vegemite at the bottom of the jar as well.
6. A dash of Worcestershire sauce, and a tablespoon of sweet chili sauce
7. Finally add salt and pepper, a generous shake of dried herbs, and a tsp of raw honey. (OK if that is not on your shelf, ordinary honey will

do.) I get my raw honey from Lithuania and pretty wonderful it is too.

8. Simmer **gently** on the stove until everything is soft, at least thirty minutes.

9. Check for taste and serve.

Pick-me-up Carrots

Ingredients:

- 1lb/500grams cooked carrots
- 2 oz butter or non-dairy margarine
- 2 tbsp honey
- ½ tsp paprika
- Juice of ½ lemon.
- Pinch salt and pepper

Method:

Stir together the carrots with all the other ingredients. in a heavy-based saucepan for five minutes until all the carrots are coated with the mixture. Serve with some chopped flat-leaved parsley sprinkled over.

This lifts carrots from extreme dullness to sparkling vivacity. It's well worth the extra trouble and calories.

Romantic Red Cabbage (because the cabbage, apples and onions get very friendly)

Ingredients:

- 1 small red cabbage (about 1lb weight.) sliced and cored.
- 2 sliced onions
- 2 eating apples
- 4 tbsp red wine or apple cider vinegar.
- 2 tbs dark brown sugar.
- Salt and pepper.
- ¼ pint water.

Method:

1. Layer the ingredients in a casserole dish, and cover with water.
2. Place in a moderate oven, (150 C.) and cook for at least an hour. This tastes even better left to cool and then reheated the next day. You could add smoked sausages to it, or diced tofu as a vegan option.

Bo Peep Pie

This is completely vegan. Bo-Peep finally realised why all her sheep ran away.

Ingredients:

- 2 tbsp vegetable oil
- 1 large, chopped onion
- 2 slim celery sticks chopped finely.
- 1 large carrot or two small ones, peeled and chopped.
- 2 chopped garlic cloves
- 1 Vegetable stock pot or two veg stock cubes.
- 1 pint of boiled water
- 3 oz brown lentils washed and drained.
- 1 large portobello mushroom, chopped into roughly 2 cm pieces.
- 1tbsp Branston pickle
- 2 tbsp tomato puree.
- 3 large potatoes or 2 potatoes and 1 sweet potato.
- Salt and pepper and dried herbs if you have some.
- 2 tbsp flora or other vegetarian margarine

Method:

1. Gently fry the onions, celery, garlic, and carrots in a thick-bottomed pan until soft. (about five minutes).
2. Add the lentils, water, tomato puree, salt and pepper, pickle, and simmer for fifteen minutes. Add the chopped mushroom and simmer everything together until most of the water is absorbed. Taste and set aside.
3. Peel and mash the potatoes until light and fluffy. You can add salt and pepper and a tbsp of English mustard if you like.
4. Place the lentil mixture into a pie dish and cover with the mashed potato. Drop little spoonsful of margarine across the surface and, fluff up the potato topping with a fork.
5. Bake at 160 for 20 minutes and serve piping hot with a green vegetable as a side dish.

Gran's Granola

This makes a delicious high-protein breakfast. Don't eat too much at once as it is very filling. Serve with the milk of your choice. The amount below will keep you going all week.

Ingredients:

- 400 grams of porridge oats, organic if possible
- 100 grams of oat bran
- 70 grams of coconut oil (about 4 tbsp)
- 3 tbsp of sunflower oil
- 150 grams of honey, or more to taste. Raw honey is best.
- ½ tsp of salt
- 2 tsp of vanilla essence
- 3 rounded tsp of ground cinnamon
- 1 tbsp of vanilla extract
- **Then add as many of the following as you have:**
  - 60 grams of ground almonds
  - 30 grams of sunflower seeds
  - 30 grams of pumpkin seeds
  - 60 grams of cashew nuts, chopped
  - 60 grams of flaked almond, lightly toasted if you prefer

- 60 grams of walnuts or pecans, chopped coarsely
- 200 grams of desiccated coconut

Method:
1. Heat oven to 150C and line two baking sheets with parchment.
2. Toss together all of the dry ingredients in a very large bowl.
3. Combine oils, honey and vanilla in a saucepan and warm over low heat until combined but below boiling point. Remove from heat and stir into dry ingredients. Mix well until everything is evenly coated with oil and honey.
4. Divided the mixture between two sheet pans and spread it evenly.
5. Bake in centre of the oven without stirring, for 20 to 30 minutes or until golden.
6. Remove from heat and allow to cool completely.
7. Take the granola off the parchment and break it apart into little clusters.
8. Store in an airtight jar or tin, or in a Ziplock bag in the fridge for several weeks.

This makes a very nice housewarming present!

High-energy mini-bites

Ingredients:

- 1 cup (8 0zs) smooth peanut butter. Don't buy any peanut butter with palm oil. There are plenty of brands that are just simply peanut butter.
- 1/3 cup of runny honey or maple syrup.
- 1 1/2 cups (or 12 oz) porridge oats
- To these add whatever you have of the following:
- 1/4 cup sunflower seeds1/4 chia seeds
- 1/2 cup of chopped, stoned dates,
- 1/2 cup desiccated coconut.
- 1/4 cup ground linseed/flax seeds. or whole if you don't have ground.
- 1/3 cup flaked almonds.
- 1 tsp vanilla
- I use Tesco's mixed seed mixture which gives even more variety. If you want to turn them into child-friendly snacks you could add some dark chocolate chips.

Method:

1. Mix all the ingredients in a large bowl and stir vigorously until everything is well combined

2. Mould into golf-ball-sized balls, and put into the fridge to set.

You can serve them in little muffin paper cases. Children and adults all love these, even though they look like something you might put on the bird table!

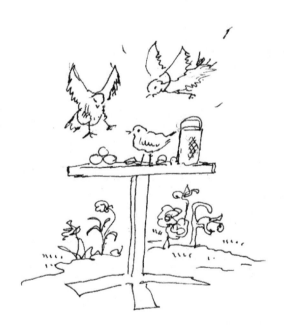

Gabriella's Stuffed Dates:

This recipe will make 10 but you can scale the ingredients up or down to your liking.

Ingredients:

10 Medjool dates

10 tsp of Peanut butter (or any other nut butter)

100g Dark chocolate

Method:

1. Remove the stones from the dates.

2. Melt the chocolate in the microwave (do this is 20 second bursts and stir in between).

3. Fill each date with 1 tsp of peanut butter.

4. Dip the dates in the melted chocolate and cover them all over.

5. Space them out on a plate in a single layer and pop them in the fridge to allow the chocolate to harden.

6. These will keep beautifully in the fridge for a few days.

Homemade Slimmer's Ice-cream

Ingredients:

- 1lb/ 500 grams of natural Yoghurt
- 1lb 500 grams of whipping cream
- 1 jar of high-fruit-content jam of choice. This could be homemade blackcurrant, strawberry, or a preserve like apricot or cherry. The Bonne Marie brand is recommended. (Jam in the USA is called Jelly.)

Method:

1. Whip the cream into stiff peaks.
2. Fold in Yoghurt
3. Gently fold in the jam until ripples appear through the whole ice cream mixture.
4. Place in a plastic box in the freezer.
5. Remove 45 mins before serving and stir vigorously. Serve in a fancy bowl.

This is still *quite* fattening of course, with the cream and jam, so serve small portions. But it contains no nasty chemical additions and looks wonderful. Everyone will be impressed and ask for your recipe!

Appendix 2

More about Jennie: What do I teach?

Combat kickboxing is a dynamic and high-intensity martial art that combines elements of traditional kickboxing with self-defence techniques. It involves striking with punches, kicks, elbows, and knees, making it a comprehensive form of combat training. Practicing combat kickboxing not only enhances physical fitness but also improves agility, coordination, and mental focus. Additionally, it provides practical self-defence skills that can be invaluable in real-life situations. Whether you're looking to improve your fitness level, boost your confidence, or learn effective self-defence techniques, combat kickboxing offers a holistic approach to personal development. With regular training, practitioners can experience increased strength, stamina, and overall well-being, making it an ideal choice for individuals seeking a challenging and rewarding martial arts discipline.

My contact details:

Website www.combatfitnesswithjennie.co.uk

All my links and a contact form are on my website.

Appendix 3

The Back of the Bus

Have you read Susanne's previous non-fiction book?

The Back of the Bus is an extraordinary account of time spent in the most remote parts of the world; staying with Apache people in New Mexico, travelling from Lake Titicaca to the islands of the Philippines, and including many times within the poorest communities across Africa. Susanne has sat with political prisoners in the overcrowded and stinking prisons of the Marcos regime, heard the stories of women who suffered torture and abuse under Pinochet, and bore witness to the worst suffering which people can endure. Yet this book is full of stories of love, hope and joy as well. It is also very funny in places.

It can be ordered as a paperback or e-book from Amazon or from the author.

"I loved this book; it is a buttress to hope over despair. Just the thing we all need right now." Anon. Reviewer.

Appendix 4

Other suggested Links and Resources

Our website:

www.feelingfightingfit.com

Our Facebook Group. -Please join us.

How to feel fighting fit with Susanne and Jennie.

Susanne also has a gardening blog, tracking her vegetable gardening adventures throughout the year. You can follow her on

mrsgarnettsgardendotcom

Appendix 5

Your Turn!

Space for your notes

_____

_____

_____

_____

_____

_____

_____

_____

_____

_____

_____

_____

_____

_____

_____

_____

_____

_____

_____

_____

_____

_____

_____

_____

_____

_____

_____

_____

_____

_____

That's all for now, folks.

Printed in Great Britain
by Amazon

38932384R00126